FUNDAMENTALS
OF CLINICAL
PSYCHOPHARMACOLOGY

D0998918

FUNDAMENTALS OF CLINICAL PSYCHOPHARMACOLOGY

Third Edition

Edited by

Ian M Anderson MA MD MRCP FRCPsych
Senior Lecturer in Psychiatry
Neuroscience and Psychiatry Unit
University of Manchester
Manchester, UK

Ian C Reid PhD MRCPsych
Professor and Head
Department of Mental Health
University of Aberdeen Medical School
Aberdeen, UK

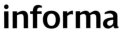

informa
healthcare

© 2006 Informa UK Ltd
First edition published in the United Kingdom in 2002 by Martin Dunitz Ltd

Second edition published in the United Kingdom in 2004 by Taylor & Francis Ltd

Third edition published in 2006 by Informa Healthcare, 4 Park Square, Milton Park, Abingdon, Oxon OX14 4RN. Informa Healthcare is a trading division of Informa UK Ltd. Registered office: 37/41 Mortimer Street, London W1T 3JH. Registered in England and Wales Number 1072954.

Tel: +44 (0)20 7017 6000
Fax: +44 (0)20 7017 6699
E-mail: info.medicine@tandf.co.uk
Website: www.informahealthcare.com

Although every effort has been made to ensure that all owners of copyright material have been acknowledged in this publication, we would be glad to acknowledge in subsequent reprints or editions any omissions brought to our attention.

Although every effort has been made to ensure that drug doses and other information are presented accurately in this publication, the ultimate responsibility rests with the prescribing physician. Neither the publishers nor the authors can be held responsible for errors or for any consequences arising from the use of information contained herein. For detailed prescribing information or instructions on the use of any product or procedure discussed herein, please consult the prescribing information or instructional material issued by the manufacturer.

A CIP record for this book is available from the British Library.

Library of Congress Cataloging-in-Publication Data

Data available on application

ISBN-10: 0 415 39565 8
ISBN-13: 978 0 415 39565 6

Distributed in North and South America by
Taylor & Francis
6000 Broken Sound Parkway, NW, (Suite 300)
Boca Raton, FL 33487, USA

Within Continental USA
Tel: 1 (800) 272 7737; Fax: 1 (800) 374 3401
Outside Continental USA
Tel: (561) 994 0555; Fax: (561) 361 6018
Email: orders@crcpress.com

Distributed in the rest of the world by
Thomson Publishing Services
Cheriton House
North Way
Andover, Hampshire SP10 5BE, UK
Tel: +44 (0)1264 332424
Email: tps.tandfsalesorder@thomson.com

Composition by J&L Composition, Filey, North Yorkshire
Printed and bound in the UK by MPG Books Ltd, Bodmin, Cornwall

Contents

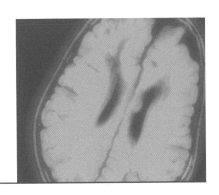

Contributors

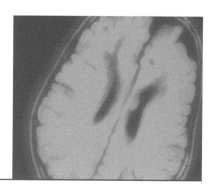

N Harry P Allen MRCPsych
Consultant Old Age Psychiatrist
Manchester Royal Infirmary
Manchester, UK

Ian M Anderson MA MD MRCP FRCPsych
Senior Lecturer in Psychiatry
Neuroscience and Psychiatry Unit
University of Manchester
Manchester, UK

David Coghill MRCPsych
Senior Lecturer and Honorary
    Consultant in Child and Adolescent
    Psychiatry
University of Dundee Department of
    Psychiatry, Centre for Child Health
Dundee, UK

Stephen J Cooper MD FRCPsych FRCPI
Senior Lecturer in Psychiatry
Division of Psychiatry and
    Neuroscience
Queen's University Belfast
Belfast, UK

Mark Daglish BSc MRCPsych
Clinical Lecturer in Psychiatry
Psychopharmacology Unit
University of Bristol, Bristol, UK

Sarah E Gartside PhD
Lecturer in Biological Psychiatry
School of Neurology, Neurobiology
    and Psychiatry
University of Newcastle
Newcastle upon Tyne, UK

Stephen M Lawrie MPhil MD MRCPsych
Senior Clinical Research Fellow
University of Edinburgh Department of
    Psychiatry
Royal Edinburgh Hospital
Edinburgh, UK

Anne Lingford-Hughes MRCPsych
Senior Lecturer in Biological
    Psychiatry and Addiction
Psychopharmacology Unit
University of Bristol
Bristol, UK

R Hamish McAllister-Williams
    BSc PhD MRCPsych
MRC Clinical Scientist Fellow
University of Newcastle
Royal Victoria Infirmary
Newcastle upon Tyne, UK

Charles A Marsden PhD
Professor of Neuropharmacology
School of Biomedical Sciences
University of Nottingham Medical
    School
Queen's Medical Centre
Nottingham, UK

Ian C Reid PhD MRCPsych
Professor, Department of Mental
    Health
University of Aberdeen Medical School
Aberdeen, UK

Michael J Travis BSc MRCPsych
Visiting Associate Professor
Western Psychiatric Institute and
    Clinic
University of Pittsburgh Medical
    Center
Pittsburgh
PA, USA
Section of Clinical
    Neuropharmacology
Division of Psychological Medicine
Institute of Psychiatry
London, UK

Allan H Young MPhil PhD FRCPsych
Professor and LEEF Chair in
    Depression Research
Associate Director of the Institute of
    Mental Health
Department of Psychiatry
University of British Columbia
Vancouver BC, Canada

Preface to the Third Edition

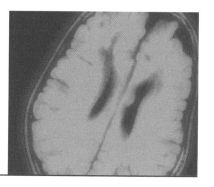

The first edition of *Fundamentals of Clinical Psychopharmacology* was published in 2002 and the second in 2004. Undertaking a third edition for 2006 would not have been possible without the enthusiasm and hard work of the authors of individual chapters, for which we are very grateful. We have also to thank the publishers for their willingness to back the relatively unusual project of updating a textbook at such short intervals, and for providing a rapid production schedule so that as far as possible the information will still be 'in-date' by publication. Our aim has been to provide more up-to-date information than is usually available in books of this kind, given the rapid developments in both basic and clinical psychopharmacology.

For this new edition, we have updated all the chapters and included a new one on the controversial topic of treating personality disorders, which has also allowed us to include rapid tranquillisation. It has been an opportunity to try to correct inevitable mistakes that creep in, and we have continued to put drug prescribing into the context of UK guidance and regulation. Since our first edition, this has increasingly become more important and is starting to have real impact on prescribing in the UK and elswhere. While it is necessary for those involved in prescribing to be aware of national guidance, it is also vital to critically evaluate the evidence and at times adopt a healthy scepticism because of the complex procedures and compromises that lie behind them.

This book is developed from the acclaimed, twice-yearly British Association for Psychopharmacology (BAP) *Psychopharmacology Course for Psychiatrists in Training*. It resulted from requests from the trainees to complement the course, and the chapters in the book reflect, and extend, the course content, ranging from basic neuroscience to the analysis of clinical trials. While it is not a comprehensive textbook of psychopharmacology, we have tried over subsequent editions to include more. We aim to provide a core of clinically relevant information about drugs in the context of current knowledge about the biological basis of the disorders that they treat. Although we have taken a UK focus in aspects of prescribing practice, the science and clinical information are international. We hope that the book will be of particular value to trainees sitting the membership examinations of the Royal College of Psychiatrists in the UK, but that it will also be useful to other clinicians, scientists and students who seek concise, up-to-date information about the field of psychopharmacology and best practice.

The current contributors to the book are leading UK psychopharmacologists, most of whom have presented the course, but we must also acknowledge the many others who have been involved in the material over the years and they are listed in the acknowledgements.

The BAP was founded in 1974, with the general intention of bringing together those from clinical and experimental disciplines as well as members of the pharmaceutical industry involved in the study of psychopharmacology. It is one of the largest national associations of its kind in the world. The BAP arranges scientific meetings, fosters research and teaching, encourages the publication of research, produces clinical guidelines, publishes the *Journal of Psychopharmacology* and provides guidance and information to the public on matters relevant to psychopharmacology. BAP evidence-based guidelines are available for downloading for personal use from our website (see below).

Membership of the BAP is open to anyone with a relevant degree related to neuroscience, including clinical medical, nursing or pharmacy degrees. If you are interested in any aspect of psychopharmacology, we would strongly encourage you to consider joining. You can find out more on our website (http://www.bap.org.uk) or contact us at:

British Association for Psychopharmacology
36 Cambridge Place
Hills Road
Cambridge CB2 1NS
UK

Ian M Anderson
Ian C Reid

Acknowledgements

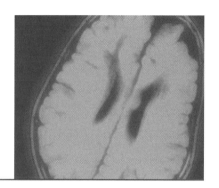

We would like to thank the following who have been involved in the development of the course material:

Dr Clive Adams
Dr David Baldwin
Dr David Balfour
Professor Thomas Barnes
Dr Geoff Bennett
Professor Philip Cowen
Professor Bill Deakin
Dr Colin Dourish
Professor Barry Everitt
Professor Nicol Ferrier
Dr Sophia Frangou
Professor Guy Goodwin
Dr Peter Haddad
Professor Chris Hollis

Dr John Hughes
Dr Eileen Joyce
Professor Robert Kerwin
Professor David King
Professor Shôn Lewis
Dr Andrea Malizia
Dr Jan Melichar
Professor David Nutt
Dr Veronica O'Keane
Dr Carmine Pariante
Dr Lyn Pilowsky
Dr Craig Ritchie
Dr Clare Stanford
Dr Stuart Watson

A Note on BANs and rINNs

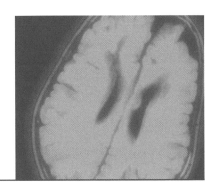

We are now required to use recommended International Non-Proprietary Names (rINNs) rather than the old British Approved Names (BANs). The name changes are mostly (but not all) minor, but it is a shame to see the loss of 'ph' to be replace by 'f' in words such as amphetamine. Adrenaline and noradrenaline alone have been retained, although dual labelling is encouraged (epinephrine and norepinephrine).

The changes became effective on 1 December 2003, with industry having up until December 2005 to finalise the name changes. Further information and a down-loadable list of drugs affected is available from the Medicines and Healthcare Products Regulatory Agency (MHRA) website: http://www.mhra.gov.uk/home/idcplg?IdcService=SS_GET_PAGE&useSecondary=true&ssDocName=CON009669

While it is likely that the old names will take time to die out, especially away from the clinical setting, we have used rINNs throughout this book, but have given both names where there might be confusion (e.g. dosulepin/dothiepin, trihexphenidyl/benzhexol).

Abbreviations

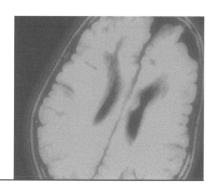

1-PP	1-pyramidinylpiperazine
2-AG	2-arachidonylglycerol
5-HIAA	5-hydroxyindoleacetic acid
5-HT	5-hydroxytryptamine, serotonin
5-HTP	5-hydroxytryptophan
5-HTPDC	5-hydroxytryptophan decarboxylase
5-HTT	5-hydroxytryptamine transporter
AC	adenylate cyclase
ACE	angiotensin-converting enzyme
ACh	acetylcholine
AChE	acetylcholinesterase
AD	Alzheimer's disease
ADAS	Alzheimer's Disease Assessment Scale
ADHD	attention deficit/hyperactivity disorder
ADL	activities of daily living
ALDH	aldehyde dehydrogenase
AMP	adenosine monophosphate
AMPA	α-amino-3-hydroxy-5-methyl-4-isoxazole propionate
AMTS	Abbreviated Mental Test Score
AP5	2-amino-5-phosphopentanoic acid
APP	amyloid precursor protein
AR	aldehyde reductase
ATP/ATPase	adenosine triphosphate/adenosine triphosphatase
AUC	area under the curve
β-CCE	ethyl-β-carboline-3-carboxylate
BDZ	benzodiazepine
BDNF	brain-derived neurotrophic factor
BNF	British National Formulary
BPSD	behavioural and psychiatric symptoms of dementia
BuChE	butyrylcholinesterase
Ca^{2+}	calcium (ion)

cAMP	cyclic adenosine monophosphate, cyclic AMP
CB	cannabinoid
CBT	cognitive–behavioural therapy
CCK	cholecystokinin
CDR	Clinical Dementia Rating
ChAT	choline acetyltransferase
CIBIC	Clinicians Interview Based Impression of Change
Cl^-	chloride (ion)
C_{max}	maximum plasma concentration (pharmacokinetics)
CNS	central nervous system
CO_2	carbon dioxide
CoA	(acetyl) coenzyme A
COMT	catechol-O-methyltransferase
C_p	plasma concentration (pharmacokinetics)
CRF	corticotropin-releasing factor
CSF	cerebrospinal fluid
CYP450	cytochrome P450
D	dopamine receptor
DA	dopamine
DAG	diacylglycerol
DAT	dopamine transporter
DβH	dopamine β-hydroxylase
DBT	dialectical behaviour therapy
DLB	dementia with Lewy bodies
DOPA	3,4-dihydroxyphenylalanine
DOPADC	DOPA decarboxylase
DOPAC	3,4-dihydroxyphenylacetic acid
DSM-IV	Fourth revision of the *Diagnostic and Statistical Manual of Mental Disease* (American Psychiatric Association)
ECG	electrocardiogram
ECS	electroconvulsive stimulation/shock (animals)
ECT	electroconvulsive therapy
EEG	electroencephalogram
EPSE	extrapyramidal side-effects
FMO	flavin-containing monooxygenase
g	gram
G	guanine nucleotide
GABA	γ-aminobutyric acid
GABA-T	GABA aminotransferase (transaminase)
GAD	glutamic acid decarboxyase (pharmacology); generalised anxiety disorder (clinical)
GDP	guanosine diphosphate
GHB	γ-hydroxybutyrate

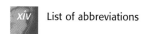

G_i	inhibitory G-protein
GIRK	G-protein-linked inward rectifying potassium channel.
G_s	stimulatory G-protein
GTP	guanosine triphosphate
H	histamine
HERG	human ether-a-gogo related gene
HPA	hypothalmic–pituitary–adrenal
HRT	hormone replacement therapy
HVA	homovanillic acid
IADL	Instrumental Activities of Daily Living
ICD-10	Tenth revision of the International Classification of Diseases (World Health Organisation)
IDDD	Interview for Deterioration in Daily Living in Dementia
IKr	delayed rectifier K^+ channel
im	intramuscular
IP_3	inositol trisphosphate
IPT	interpersonal therapy
ITT	intention-to-treat
K^+	potassium
LAAM	levo-α-acetylmethadol
LC	locus coeruleus
LOCF	last observation carried forward
LSD	lysergic acid diethylamide
LTA	lateral tegmental area
LTP	long-term potentiation
M	muscarinic
MAO	monoamine oxidase
MAOI	monoamine oxidase inhibitor
MDA	methylenedioxyamfetamine (Adam)
MDD	major depressive disorder
MDEA	methylenedioxyethylamfetamine (Eve)
MDMA	methylenedioxymethamfetamine (Ecstasy)
mg	milligram
Mg^{2+}	magnesium
MGluR	metabotropic glutamate receptor
MHPG	3-methoxy-4-hydroxyphenylethylene glycol
MHRA	Medicines and Healthcare products Regulatory Authority (UK)
mL	millilitre
mmol/L	millimoles/litre
MK-801	dizocilpine
MMRM	mixed effects model repeated measures

MMSE	Mini-Mental State Examination
MOUSEPAD	Manchester and Oxford Universities Scale for the Psychopathological Assessment of Dementia
MT	methoxytyramine
NA	noradrenaline
Na$^+$	sodium ion
NAcc	nucleus accumbens
NARI	noradrenaline reuptake inhibitor
NaSSa	noradrenaline- and serotonin-specific antidepressant
NAT	noradrenaline transporter
NICE	National Institute for (Health and) Clinical Excellence (UK)
NK	neurokinin
NMDA	N-methyl D-aspartate
NM	normetanephrine
NMS	neuroleptic malignant syndrome
NPI	Neuropsychiatric Inventory
NPY	neuropeptide Y
NSAID	nonsteroidal anti-inflammatory drug
NT	neurotensin
OCD	obsessive–compulsive disorder
OX	orexin
PAG	periaqueductal grey
PCP	phencyclidine (Angel Dust)
pCPA	p-chlorophenylalanine
PEM	prescription event monitoring
PET	positron emission tomography
PFC	prefrontal cortex
pH	negative logarithm of hydrogen ion concentration (measure of acidity/alkalinity)
PKC	protein kinase C
PLC	phospholipase C
PNMT	phenylethanolamine-N-methyltransferase
PTSD	post-traumatic stress disorder
Q	quantity of drug (pharmacokinetics)
QTc	interval between Q and T waves on the electrocardiogram corrected for heart rate
RCT	randomised controlled trial
RIMA	reversible inhibitor of monoamine oxidase A
RT	rapid tranquillisation
SERT	serotonin (5-HT) transporter, 5-HTT

SNRI	serotonin and noradrenaline reuptake inhibitor
SPECT	single photon emission computed tomography
SSRI	selective serotonin reuptake inhibitor
$t_{1/2}$	half-life (pharmacokinetics)
TCAs	tricyclic antidepressants
THA	tacrine, tetrahydroaminoacridine
THC	Δ^9-tetrahydrocannabinol
t_{max}	time to maximum (peak) plasma concentration
TPH	tryptopham hydroxylase
TRH	thyrotropin-releasing hormone
UDPGT	uridine diphosphate glucuronosyltransferase
V_d	volume of distribution (pharmacokinetics)
VMA	vanillylmandelic acid
VNTR	variable number tandem repeat (e.g. polymorphism of 5-HTT)
VTA	ventral tegmental area

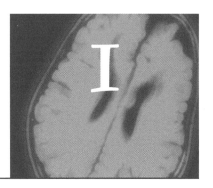

Neuropharmacology and drug action

Sarah E Gartside and Charles A Marsden

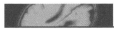 ## Introduction

This chapter will concentrate on neurotransmission and the mechanisms by which psychotropic drugs relevant to the treatment of psychiatric disorders alter neurotransmission.

- Most drugs used in psychiatry, as well as nontherapeutic psychotropic drugs, act to alter neurotransmission.
- In general, drugs act either *presynaptically* to influence levels of the neurotransmitter in the synaptic cleft or *postsynaptically* by agonist, antagonist or modulatory actions at postsynaptic receptors.

 ## Neurotransmission

Neurotransmission describes the process by which information is transferred from one neuron to another neuron (or other cell type) across the synaptic cleft (Fig. 1.1). It involves:

- release of a neurotransmitter from the presynaptic nerve ending in response to the arrival of an action potential.
- subsequent activation of a receptor on the membrane of the postsynaptic neuron.

Activation of the postsynaptic receptor may result in either:

- *excitation* – membrane depolarisation, or
- *inhibition* – membrane hyperpolarisation.

These membrane effects may be due to either:

- a direct effect on an ion channel (*fast neurotransmission*; Fig. 1.2), or
- an indirect effect via a guanine nucleotide-binding (G)-protein to cause the opening of ion channels or the stimulation or inhibition of an enzyme and

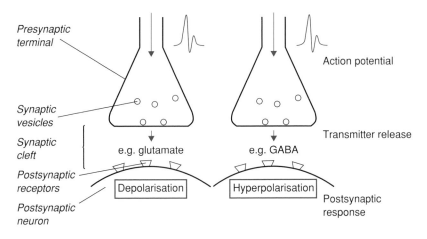

Figure 1.1 Synaptic transmission involves release of a neurotransmitter from the presynaptic nerve ending and its binding to a postsynaptic receptor to produce a change in function (excitation or inhibition) in the postsynaptic neuron.
GABA, γ-aminobutyric acid.

consequent increase or decrease in a second messenger (*slow neurotransmission*; Fig. 1.2) (see 'Receptor mechanisms' below).

The initial receptor response (i.e. excitation or inhibition) does not necessarily describe the final functional output; for example, inhibition of an inhibitory neuron will cause disinhibition of the next neuron in the chain and thus a net excitatory response (see Fig. 7.1 for an example). Behaviour is thus the result of a complex interplay between many neurons, and it is therefore very difficult to explain a particular behaviour as being the result of the action of a single neurotransmitter.

Coexistence of neurotransmitters

▪ The major neurotransmitters in the brain are noradrenaline (NA, also called norepinephrine), dopamine (DA), 5-hydroxytryptamine (5-HT, also called serotonin), acetylcholine (ACh), glutamate and γ-aminobutyric acid (GABA).
▪ The original concept of chemical neurotransmission posited that only one active substance (neurotransmitter) was released from the presynaptic terminal.
▪ This has been modified to incorporate the idea of cotransmission, when two or more biologically active substances are released in response to an action potential.
▪ However, all the substances released do not necessarily act as neurotransmitters (i.e. produce a functional response in the postsynaptic neuron).
▪ Some substances released from nerve endings act as neuromodulators (i.e.

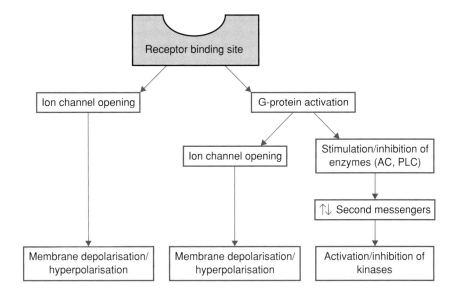

Figure 1.2   Fast neurotransmission mediated by ligand-gated ion channel receptors (e.g. the glutamate NMDA (*N*-methyl-D-aspartate) receptor and the γ-aminobutyric acid receptor) involves direct opening of an ion channel, while slow neurotransmission mediated through G-protein-coupled receptors (e.g. the dopamine D_2 receptor and the serotonin 5-HT$_{1A}$ receptor) involves indirect ion channel opening or second-messenger production/inhibition. Activation of kinase enzymes by the second messengers cAMP and diacylglycerol (DAG) leads to changes in intracellular processes, including ion transport and enzyme activity. AC, adenylate cyclase; PLC, phospholipase C.

interact with the neurotransmitter to either facilitate or reduce its action without causing functional effects of their own).

▦ Amine neurotransmitters – DA, NA, 5-HT and ACh – commonly coexist with various neuropeptides, e.g. cholecystokinin (CCK), neurotensin (NT) and thyrotropin-releasing hormone (TRH), which act as either:
 – full neurotransmitters (i.e. produce a functional response on their own), or
 – neuromodulators (when they modulate the responsiveness of the amine neurotransmitter).

▦ Coexistence is probably the normal state of affairs, although there is little detailed understanding of its functional importance or about the ways in which it could impact on drug treatment.

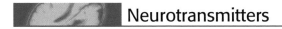 # Neurotransmitters

Table 1.1 lists the major neurotransmitters in the brain, together with the functions and neurological/psychiatric disorders in which they are thought to play a role. Some of the other neurotransmitters/neuromodulators and in particular some of the numerous neuropeptides found in the brain are also given.

Table 1.1 Central nervous system neurotransmitters and neuromodulators: the major neurotransmitters and neuromodulators together with the functions and disorders with which they are associated

Class	Neurorotransmitter	Function/disorder
Amines	Acetylcholine (ACh)	Alzheimer's disease
	Dopamine (DA)	Parkinson's disease, schizophrenia
	Noradrenaline (NA)	Anxiety, depression, cognition, schizophrenia,
	5-Hydroxytryptamine	Depression, anxiety/panic/OCD, schizophrenia
	(5-HT, serotonin)	Alzheimer's disease, migraine, hallucinations, eating disorders
	Histamine	Arousal, cognition
Amino acids	Glutamate	Neurodegeneration
	γ-Aminobutyric acid (GABA)	Anxiety, Huntington's disease
Peptides	Met/Leu-enkephalin	Pain, mood
	β-Endorphin	Pain, mood
	Substance P/tachykinins	Huntington's disease, depression
	Vasopressin	Cognition
	Cholecystokinin (CCK)	Anxiety, pain
	Neurotensin (NT)	Schizophrenia
	Thyrotropin-releasing hormone (TRH)	Arousal, motorneuron disease
	Neuropeptide Y (NPY)	Feeding
	Corticotropin-releasing factor (CRF)	Anxiety, depression
	Orexins	Circadian function, feeding, response to stress
Other	Endocannabinoids	Pain, schizophrenia, eating disorders

▨ To date, over 60 neuropeptides have been identified; the best understood are the enkephalins, which activate opioid receptors.

▨ The neurokinins (substance P, neurokinin A and neurokinin B) and their receptors (NK_1, NK_2 and NK_3) have recently attracted interest as possible targets for antidepressant and antipsychotic drugs.

▨ Neurotensin (NT) has been postulated as a possible target for treating schizophrenia because of its coexistence with DA and its ability to modulate DA-induced behaviours.

▨ CCK administration can induce panic attacks (especially in panic disorder patients), possibly involving both brain and peripheral mechanisms. However, CCK receptor antagonists have not been successful anti-panic drugs but this may in part relate to poor brain penetration of the compounds.

▨ Corticotropin-releasing factor (CRF) receptor (CRF_1, CRF_2) antagonists are currently under clinical evaluation as antidepressants and anxiolytics.

- Orexins A and B (hypocretins) are closely related neuropeptides derived from a single gene. They act on OX_1 and OX_2 receptors, which are highly expressed in the lateral hypothalamus and other brain areas involved in stress regulation. Orexins were initially identified as important regulators of feeding, but are now also seen as involved in circadian function, sleep and response to stress, including neuroendocrine control.
- Anandamide is one of several endogenous agonists of cannabinoid type 1 (CB_1) and type 2 (CB_2) receptors. CB_1 receptors are found in the brain and are potential targets for the treatment of pain and various mood disorders. CB_2 receptors are associated with the immune system.
- Neurosteroids (i.e. steroids made within the brain) and steroids with access to the brain interact with steroid receptors and also modulate the function of $GABA_A$ receptors and are thus potential anti-anxiety drug targets (see Chapter 6).
- Various neurotrophic factors also have an important role not only in the normal development of the brain, but also in maintaining synaptic function (and in some cases regulating transmitter release) in the adult brain. An example is brain-derived neurotrophic factor (BDNF), the expression of which is increased by chronic antidepressant treatment in animals and so may be involved in the mechanism of action of these drugs.

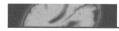

Organisation of neurotransmitter pathways

The major neurotransmitter pathways – and those most important in psychopharmacology – can be divided organisationally into three groups:

- Long ascending and descending axonal pathways derived from discrete neuronal cell groups located within specific brain nuclei. This organisation is a feature of catecholamine (DA, NA) and indoleamine (5-HT) as well as many cholinergic (ACh) pathways (Fig 1.3).
- Long and short axonal pathways derived from neuronal cell bodies widely distributed throughout the brain. The major excitatory (glutamate) and inhibitory (GABA) neurotransmitters are organised in this way.
- Short intraregional pathways within the cerebral cortex, striatum, etc. Many of these so-called 'interneurons' are GABAergic, but various neuropeptide neurons (e.g. somatostatin neurons in the cerebral cortex) are also organised in this way.

Receptor mechanisms

The main targets for psychotropic drug action are receptors and transporters. Receptors for neurotransmitters are located on membranes and are:

- directly coupled to an ion channel (ligand-gated ion channel or *ionotropic* receptors), and mediate fast neurotransmission (e.g. *N*-methyl-D-aspartate (NMDA)-type glutamate receptor, $GABA_A$ and nicotinic ACh receptors); or

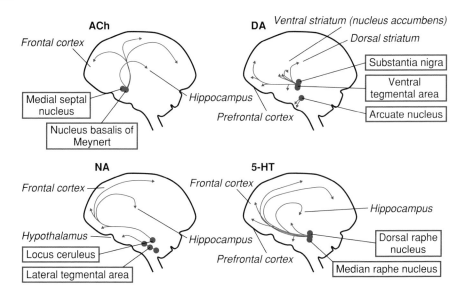

Figure 1.3 Diagram of the main pathways of cholinergic (ACh), dopaminergic (DA), noradrenergic (NA) and serotonergic (5-HT) neurons in the brain. Note the discrete localisation of the neuronal cell bodies and the long ascending projections.

▪ coupled to an intracellular effector system via a G-protein (also called *metabotropic* receptors), and mediate slow neurotransmission (e.g. DA, NA, most 5-HT and muscarinic ACh receptors).

Ligand-gated ion channel receptors

▪ Ligand-gated ion channel receptors consist of four or five protein subunits arranged to form a central channel or pore.
▪ Binding of the transmitter (or other agonist) to the receptor causes a conformational change in the proteins that results in opening of the channel, allowing specific ions to pass through.
▪ Ion channel opening occurs in milliseconds; thus there are rapid excitatory or inhibitory effects, depending on which ion(s) the channel is permeable to.

G-protein receptors (Fig. 1.4)

▪ G-protein receptors are so named because their action is linked to the binding of guanine nucleotide-binding (G)-protein.
▪ They consist of a protein that crosses the membrane seven times, with loops inside and outside the cell. One of the internal loops is larger than the rest and interacts with the G-protein.

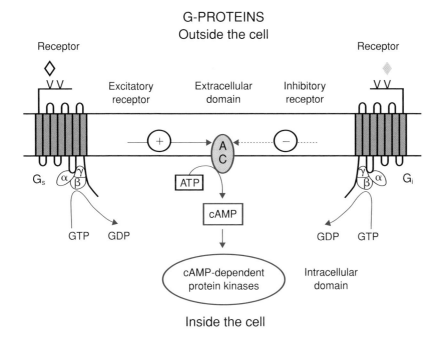

Figure 1.4   G-proteins couple the receptor binding site to the second-messenger system; they consist of three subunits (α, β, γ) anchored to the seven transmembrane helices that form the receptor. Coupling of the α subunit to an agonist-occupied receptor causes bound guanosine diphosphate (GDP) to exchange with guanosine triphosphate (GTP), and the resulting α–GTP complex leaves the receptor to interact with a target protein (an enzyme such as adenylate cyclase (AC) or an ion channel). There is then hydrolysis of the bound GTP to GDP, and the α subunit links again to the βγ subunit. The G-protein mechanism can be either inhibitory (G_i) or excitatory (G_s). In summary, the G-proteins provide the link between the ligand-recognition site and the effector system.
ATP, adenosine triphosphate; cAMP, cyclic adenosine monophosphate.

- The G-protein has three subunits (α, β, γ), with the α unit containing guanosine triphosphatase (GTPase) activity.
- When the transmitter or agonist binds to the receptor, α–guanosine triphosphate (α–GTP) is released, which then can either activate or inhibit one of two major second-messenger systems:
  - *Adenylate cyclase/cyclic adenosine monophosphate (cAMP)*. cAMP, which is produced by the enzyme adenylate cyclase, activates various protein kinases, which in turn influence the function of various enzymes, carriers, etc. Receptors can be either positively or negatively coupled to adenylate cyclase, causing stimulation (excitation) or inhibition of the enzyme, respectively (Fig. 1.4).
  - *Phospholipase C (PLC)/inositol trisphosphate (IP_3)/diacylglycerol (DAG)*. Activation of the enzyme PLC results in the formation of two intracellular

messengers: IP_3 and DAG. IP_3 increases free calcium (Ca^{2+}), thus activating various enzymes. DAG activates protein kinase C (PKC), which in turn regulates various intracellular functions.

- G-proteins can also control potassium (K^+) and Ca^{2+} channel function, thus regulating membrane excitability and transmitter release; e.g. 5-HT_{1A} receptor activation inhibits adenylate cyclase and increases K^+ conductance, causing hyperpolarisation.

Some examples of receptor types

- The NMDA and α-amino-3-hydroxy-5-methyl-4-isoxazole propionate (AMPA) receptors for glutamate are ligand-gated ion channels that mediate fast-acting excitatory neurotransmission through the opening of sodium (Na^+) channels. 5-HT_3 and nicotinic ACh receptors are also excitatory ligand-gated ion channels.
- The $GABA_A$ receptor is linked to a chloride (Cl^-) channel and mediates fast inhibitory neurotransmission. Binding of the transmitter GABA to the receptor results in an influx of Cl^- into the neuron, causing hyperpolarisation (see Fig 1.11). The glycine receptor is also an inhibitory ligand-gated ion channel.
- Many of the receptors for the amine neurotransmitters (DA, NA, 5-HT) as well as muscarinic ACh receptors are G-protein-linked:
  - 5-HT_{1A}, $GABA_B$, M_2 (muscarinic ACh) receptors and α_2-adrenoceptors are linked via a G-protein to inhibition of adenylate cyclase. These receptors can also be linked via the G-protein to Ca^{2+} and K^+ channels. Receptor activation causes a decrease in Ca^{2+} conductance and an increase in K^+ conductance, and results in hyperpolarisation.
  - 5-HT_7 receptors and β_1- and β_2-adrenoceptors are linked via a G-protein to stimulation of adenylate cyclase.
  - α_1-adrenoceptors and M_1 (muscarinic ACh) and 5-HT_2 receptors are linked via a G-protein to stimulation of PLC.

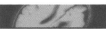 Receptor location

- The location of a receptor determines its effects on neurotransmission (Fig. 1.5).
- Receptors are mostly located on a membrane on the far side of the synaptic cleft to the point of neurotransmitter release. These postsynaptic receptors may be located on:
  - dendrites or the soma of a neuron, in which case they regulate cell firing; or
  - a nerve terminal, in which case the function will be to regulate neurotransmitter release; in this situation the receptor is sometimes referred to as a *presynaptic heteroceptor*.
- Receptors located on the same type of neuron that releases the neurotransmitter that activates it are termed *autoreceptors* and are concerned with the

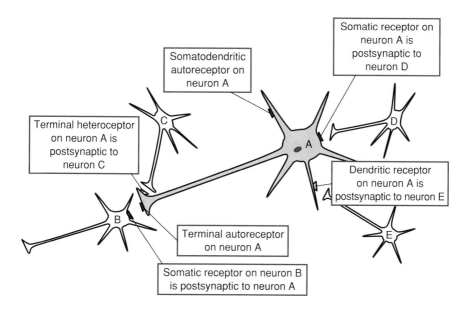

Figure 1.5 Nomenclature used to describe receptor location on neurons. Starting with 'neuron A', neurotransmitter released at the terminals will interact with **postsynaptic** receptors on 'neuron B'. Similarly, neurotransmitter released from 'neurons D and E' will interact with postsynaptic receptor on 'neuron A'. Neurotransmitter released from 'neuron A' will also regulate its own release by interacting with the **terminal autoreceptor** or affect neuronal firing by interacting with the **somatodendritic autoreceptor**. Release of neurotransmitter from 'neuron A' can also be regulated by activation of **presynaptic heteroceptors** on the terminals, which are postsynaptic receptors activated by neurotransmitter from 'neuron C'.

autoregulation (normally inhibitory feedback). Autoreceptors located on the soma or dendrites of the neuron are termed *somatodendritic autoreceptors* and regulate neuronal firing. Autoreceptors located on the presynaptic terminal are called *terminal autoreceptors* and regulate release.

- The DA autoreceptor at both sites is the D_2 receptor; similarly, the NA autoreceptor is the α_2-adrenoceptor; and M_2 muscarinic receptors act as somatodendritic and terminal autoreceptors on cholinergic neurons. In the case of 5-HT neurons, the somatodendritic autoreceptor is of the 5-HT$_{1A}$ subtype, while the terminal autoreceptors are of the 5-HT$_{1B}$ or 5-HT$_{1D}$ subtypes.

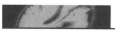 ## Neurotransmitter transporters

Transporters are a second major target for psychotropic drugs:

- Most neurotransmitters are removed from the synaptic cleft by high-affinity transporters.

▦   This process terminates their action on postsynaptic and presynaptic receptors.

▦   The neurotransmitter transporters are a family of single protein chains that cross the neuronal membrane 12 times.

▦   Neurotransmitter transporters are actually cotransporters transporting Na^+ ions into the cell. It is the concentration gradient for Na^+ that drives the transport of the neurotransmitter. Because Na^+ ions are transported along with the neurotransmitter, neurotransmitter transporters are electrogenic.

▦   There is high sequence homology between transporters for DA (DAT), NA (NAT) and 5-HT (SERT, or 5-HTT). This means that some drugs have poor selectivity between transporters; e.g. tricyclic antidepressants block both 5-HTT and NAT.

▦   Amfetamines gain entry to nerve terminals via the transporter. The neurotransmitter selectivity of the various amfetamine derivatives – e.g. methylenedioxymethamfetamine (MDMA, Ecstasy) (affecting 5-HT, NA and DA), methamfetamine (affecting DA) and fenfluramine (affecting 5-HT) – is determined by their affinity for the particular transporter. Once inside the terminal, these drugs cause release of neurotransmitter, which is independent of depolarisation (i.e. of a nerve impulse).

▦   Some monoamine neurotoxins (e.g. 6-hydroxydopamine) also access nerve terminals via the transporter.

▦   There are four known types of GABA transporter, with different structure, distribution and pharmacology.

▦   Inhibitors of GABA transport (e.g. tiagabine) have anticonvulsant activity.

▦   To date, inhibitors of glutamate transport have no therapeutic use.

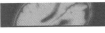 Dopamine (DA)

Pathways and functions

DA-containing neuronal cell bodies are located in three discrete areas (Fig. 1.3):

▦   *Substantia nigra*: axons project from this midbrain area to the basal ganglia (dorsal striatum, caudate–putamen).
 –   They are involved in the initiation of motor plans and motor coordination, and this pathway is the primary site of degeneration in Parkinson's disease.
 –   Antipsychotic drugs (D_2-receptor antagonists) produce motor disturbances by blocking D_2 receptors in the caudate–putamen).

▦   *Ventral tegmental area* (VTA): axons project to the nucleus accumbens (ventral striatum), amygdala and prefrontal cortex. These are referred to as the mesolimbic and mesocortical DA pathways. They are strongly associated with motivation, reward behaviour and drug dependence. Many drugs of abuse increase DA transmission in these pathways; e.g. amfetamines cause DA release, cocaine blocks DA reuptake, and opioids, cannabinoids and nicotine all increase the firing of DA neurons (see Chapter 7). These pathways are also considered important in schizophrenia and an important site of action for antipsychotic drugs (D_2 and D_4 antagonists).

▓ *Tuberoinfundibular DA pathway*: neurones in the arcuate nucleus project into the median eminence and release DA in the hypophyseal portal system. DA inhibits prolactin release from the anterior pituitary via activation of D_2 receptors. Drugs that block D_2 receptors (e.g. antipsychotics) increase prolactin secretion, causing gynaecomastia, galactorrhoea and amenorrhoea.

Synthesis and metabolism (Table 1.2, Fig. 1.6)

▓ DA is synthesised from the amino acid tyrosine by the actions of the enzymes tyrosine hydroxylase and DOPA decarboxylase. Tyrosine is first hydroxylated to form the intermediate 3,4-dihydroxyphenylanine (DOPA), which is in turn decarboxylated to form DA. Tyrosine hydroxylase is inhibited by α-methyl-*p*-tyrosine.

Table 1.2 Neurotransmitter synthesis and metabolism: summary of the enzymes involved in the synthesis and metabolism of amine and amino acid neurotransmitters

Transmitter	Precursor	Synthetic enzymes	Inactivation
Acetylcholine (ACh)	Choline Acetyl CoA	ChAT	Extracellular AChE Choline taken up and recycled
Dopamine (DA)	Tyrosine	TH (to DOPA) DOPADC (to DA)	Reuptake followed by metabolism by MAO-B and COMT
Noradrenaline (NA)	Tyrosine	TH (to DOPA) DOPADC (to DA) DβH (to NA)	Reuptake followed by metabolism by MAO-A and COMT
Serotonin (5-HT)	Tryptophan	TPH (to 5-HTP) 5-HTPDC (to 5-HT)	Reuptake followed by metabolism by MAO-A
Glutamate	Glutamine	Glutaminase	Reuptake followed by metabolism by GAD (GABA shunt)
GABA	Glutamate	GAD	Reuptake followed by metabolism by GABA-T

AChE, acetylcholinesterase; ChAT, choline acetyltransferase; COMT, catechol-*O*-methyltransferase; DβH, dopamine-β-hydroxylase; DA, dopamine; DOPA, 3,4-dihydroxyphenylalanine; DOPADC, DOPA decarboxylase; GABA-T, GABA aminotransferase (transaminase); GAD, glutamic acid decarboxylase; 5-HTP, 5-hydroxytryptophan; 5-HTPDC, 5-HTP decarboxylase; MAO, monoamine oxidase; TH, tyrosine hydroxylase; TPH, tryptophan hydroxylase.

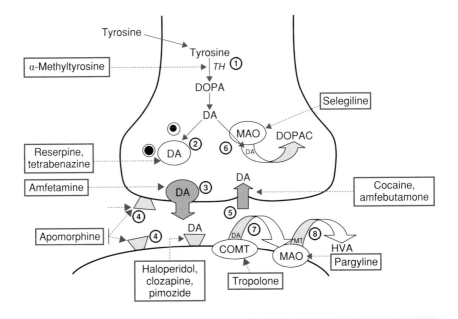

Figure 1.6 Schematic model of a central dopaminergic terminal, indicating possible sites of drug action. Tyrosine hydroxylase activity, and hence dopamine (DA) synthesis, are blocked by the irreversible competitive inhibitor, α-methyltyrosine, preventing the synthesis of 3,4-dihydroxyphenylalanine (DOPA) (1). Reserpine and tetrabenazine interfere with the uptake-storage mechanism of the amine granules. The depletion of DA produced by reserpine is long-lasting, and the storage granules appear to be irreversibly damaged. Tetrabenazine also intereferes with the uptake storage mechanism of the granules, but the effects of this drug do not appear to be irreversible (2). Amfetamine enters the terminal via the dopamine reuptake transporter DAT (5) and releases DA from the vesicles (3). Apomorphine is a nonselective DA receptor agonist with both pre- and postsynaptic sites of action. Haloperidol, pimozide, clozapine and other antipsychotics are D_2-receptor antagonists (4). Released DA has its action terminated by reuptake into presynaptic terminal. Cocaine and amfebutamone (bupropion) are inhibitors of this reuptake mechanism (5). DA present in the cytosol of the presynaptic terminal can be degraded by the enzyme monoamine oxidase (MAO), which is located in the outer membrane of the mitochondria (6). 3,4-Dihydroxyphenylacetic acid (DOPAC) is a product of the action of MAO and aldehyde dehydrogenase on DA. Selegiline is an inhibitor of MAO-B. DA can also be inactivated to methoxytyramine (MT) by the enzyme catechol-O-methyl transferase (COMT), which is believed to be localised outside the presynaptic neuron. Tropolone is an inhibitor of COMT (7). Some MAO is also present outside the dopaminergic neuron (8), where it metabolises MT to homovanillic acid (HVA).

- The transmitter is stored in vesicles, where it is protected from degradation by monoamine oxidase (MAO).
- Following release, DA is taken back up into the presynaptic terminal by the DA transporter.
- DA is metabolised by mitochondrial MAO (mainly MAO-B) and membrane-bound enzyme catechol-O-methyltransferase (COMT) to form DOPAC homovanillic acid (HVA).

■ Both MAO and COMT inhibitors are used in the symptomatic treatment of Parkinson's disease.
■ DA release is under inhibitory autoreceptor feedback regulation by the presynaptic D_2 and/or D_3 dopamine receptors; activation of these receptors results in inhibition of DA release.

DA receptors (Table 1.3)

■ Five DA receptors have been identified using pharmacological and molecular biological methods.
■ There are two families: the 'D_1-like' family comprising D_1 and D_5 receptors, which are positively coupled to adenylate cyclase; and the 'D_2-like' (D_2, D_3, D_4), which are negatively coupled to adenylate cyclase.

Table 1.3 Dopamine receptors: distribution, function, signal transduction and pharmacology of dopamine receptors in the brain

		D_1-like		D_2-like[a]		
		D_1	D_5	D_2	D_3	D_4
Distribution	*Functional role*					
Cortex	Arousal, mood	++	–	++	–	–
Limbic system	Emotion, stereotypical behaviour	+++	–	+++	+	++
Basal ganglia	Motor control	++	+	+++	+	+
Hypothalamus	Autonomic and endocrine control	++	+	–	–	–
Pituitary gland	Endocrine control	–	–	+++	–	–
Signal transduction		Increase cAMP		Decrease cAMP		
Agonists:						
Dopamine		+(low potency)		+(high potency)		
Bromocriptine		Partial agonist				
Antagonists:						
Chlorpromazine		+	+	+++	+++	+
Haloperidol		++	+	+++	+++	+++
Clozapine		+	+	+	+	++
Effect		Postsynaptic inhibition		Pre- and postsynaptic inhibition		

[a] There are short and long forms of D_2 receptors and variants of D_3 and D_4.
cAMP, cyclic adenosine monophosphate.
–, not functionally involved; +, ++, +++, slightly, moderately, very, functionally involved respectively

- There are further variants, with short and long forms of the D_2 receptor, and genetic polymorphisms (D_4 in particular).
- Both D_1 and D_2 receptors have wide distribution (striatal, mesolimbic and hypothalamic), while D_3 and D_4 are more localised.
- The D_2 receptor is found both on DA neurons (as a somatodendritic and terminal autoreceptor) and at postsynaptic sites, so D_2 antagonists not only inhibit postsynaptic responses but also increase DA release by antagonism of the autoreceptor.
- Both typical and atypical antipsychotics have high affinity for D_2 receptors. The atypical antipsychotic clozapine has a high affinity for the D_4 receptor, which may be important in its distinct clinical profile.

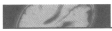 Noradrenaline (NA)

Pathways and functions (Fig 1.3)

- The principal location of the soma of NA-containing neurons is the locus ceruleus (LC), with the axons projecting up to limbic areas (via the dorsal noradrenergic bundle) and descending to the spinal cord (involved in muscle coordination). Nuclei in the lateral tegmental area (LTA) of the medulla also contain noradrenergic cell bodies. Projections from the LTA innervate forebrain regions via the ventral noradrenergic bundle.
- LC and LTA neurons project to the hypothalamus, cortex and subcortical limbic areas.
- The cortical projections are concerned with arousal and maintaining the cortex in an alert state. The limbic projections are involved in drive, motivation, mood and response to stress.

Synthesis and metabolism (Table 1.2, Fig 1.7)

- NA is synthesised from tyrosine by the enzymes tyrosine hydroxylase and DOPA decarboxylase (see under DA above). The resulting DA is converted to NA by the action of dopamine-β-hydroxylase, which is found exclusively in noradrenergic and adrenergic neurons.
- NA is stored in vesicles protected from MAO and ready for release in response to terminal depolarisation.
- The action of released NA on receptors is terminated by reuptake; a process inhibited by tricyclic antidepressants, reboxetine, venlafaxine and duloxetine, as well as cocaine.
- NA, like DA, is metabolised by MAO (mainly MAO-A) and COMT. The main CNS metabolite of NA is 3-methoxy-4-hydroxyphenylethylene glycol (MHPG). This is in contrast to the periphery, where the main metabolite is vanillylmandelic acid (VMA).
- NA release is under inhibitory feedback regulation by α_2-autoreceptors.

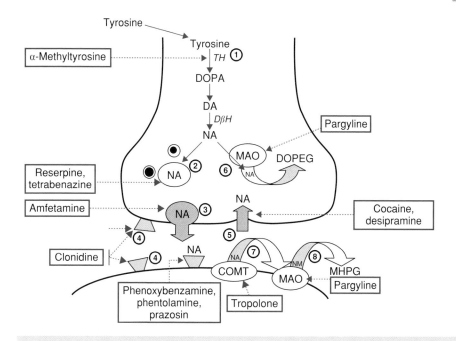

Figure 1.7 Schematic model of central noradrenergic terminal, indicating possible sites of drug action. Tyrosine hydroxylase can be blocked by α-methyltyrosine, preventing synthesis of 3,4-dihydroxyphenylalamine (DOPA), while dopamine-β-hydroxylase (DβH) activity is blocked by disulfiram (1). Reserpine and tetrabenazine interfere with the synaptic vesicles, preventing storage of the transmitter. The depletion of noradrenaline (NA) produced by reserpine is long-lasting, and the storage vesicles are irreversibly damaged. Tetrabenazine also interferes with the uptake and/or storage mechanism, but the effects are reversible (2). Amfetamine causes release of NA from the vesicles after entering the terminal via the reuptake transporter (3). Receptors are located on the presynaptic terminal (α_2-autoreceptors) and on the postsynaptic neuron (α_1, α_2, β_1, β_2). Clonidine, an α_2-receptor agonist, reduces NA release by stimulating autoreceptors. Yohimbine and piperoxane are selective α_2-antagonists. Phenoxybenzamine and phentolamine are α_1-receptor antagonists (4). NA has its action terminated by uptake. The uptake transporter is blocked by tricyclic antidepressants (TCAs) such as desipramine, as well as by reboxetine, venlafaxine and duloxetine and by cocaine (5). NA in the cytosol of the terminal is vulnerable to degradation by the enzyme monoamine oxidase (MAO) to an intermediate aldelyde product that is then reduced by aldehyde reductase (AR) to 3,4-dihydroxyphenylethylene glycol (DOPEG). Pargyline is an effective inhibitor of MAO (6). NA can be inactivated to normetanephrine (NM) by the membrane-bound enzyme catechol-*O*-methyltransferase (COMT) (7). Tropolone is an inhibitor of COMT. The normetanephrine (NM) formed by the action of COMT on NA can be further metabolised by MAO and AR to 3-methoxy-4-hydroxyphenylethylene glycol (MHPG) (8).

Adrenoceptors

The receptors on which noradrenaline acts are divided into α- and β-adrenoceptors, with further subdivisions within these two main groups.

- Both α_1- and α_2-adrenoreceptors are found within the brain at postsynaptic sites. The α_2 adrenoceptor is also located on noradrenergic terminals and noradrenergic cell bodies, where it acts as the autoreceptor.
- α_1-adrenoceptors are excitatory and use inositol phosphate as the second messenger. α_2-adrenoceptors are inhibitory and are negatively linked to adenylate cyclase (i.e. they inhibit cAMP production). Clonidine is an α_2-adrenoceptor agonist, which is used in the management of morphine withdrawal. It is believed to act presynaptically to reduce NA release, which is increased during withdrawal.
- β-adrenoceptors (β_1, β_2, β_3) are stimulatory and positively linked to adenylate cyclase (i.e. they increase cAMP). Antagonists of β-adrenoceptors (β-blockers) are used in the treatment of anxiety – particularly performance anxiety. It is thought that they act both centrally and peripherally to reduce autonomic symptoms.

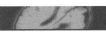 Serotonin (5-hydroxytryptamine, 5-HT)

Pathways and functions (Fig 1.3)

- The cell bodies of neurons containing 5-HT are located in the midbrain and brainstem raphe nuclei, from which there extend long ascending (dorsal and median raphe) or descending (obscurus, magnus and pallidus raphe nuclei) pathways.
- The ascending pathways innervate many forebrain regions, including the hippocampus, striatum, amygdala and hypothalamus, and cerebral cortex. The terminal fields of dorsal and median raphe projections overlap, but some regions have predominantly dorsal raphe (e.g. frontal cortex) or median raphe (e.g. dorsal hippocampus) derived innervation. 5-HT has a modulatory role in various aspects of behaviour, including mood and emotion, sleep/ wakefulness and regulation of circadian functions, control of feeding and sexual behaviours, body temperature, perceptions, and emesis.
- The descending pathways terminate in the dorsal horn of the spinal cord – where they are involved in the inhibition of pain transmission – and the ventral horn – where they regulate motorneuron output.

Synthesis and metabolism (Table 1.2, Fig 1.8)

- 5-HT is formed from the amino acid tryptophan, by the action of the enzymes tryptophan hydroxylase, and 5-HTP decarboxylase. The intermediate in 5-HT synthesis is 5-hydroxytryptophan (5-HTP).
- Tryptophan hydroxylase is the rate-limiting enzyme in the synthesis of 5-HT, and importantly, is unsaturated by the normal concentrations of tryptophan in

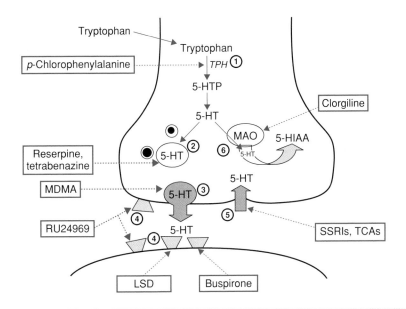

Figure 1.8 Schematic model of a central serotonergic terminal, indicating possible sites of drug action. Tryptophan is converted to 5-hydroxytryptophan (5-HTP) by tryptophan hydroxylase (TPH) (1), and this enzyme can be inhibited by p-chlorophenylalanine (pCPA). 5-HTP is then converted to 5-HT and stored in vesicles (2) protected from degradation by monoamine oxidase (MAO). The vesicles can be disrupted by reserpine and tetrabenazine. p-Chloroamfetamine, fenfluramine and methylenedioxymethamfetamine (MDMA, Ecstasy) can enter 5-HT terminals via the transporter and cause the release of the transmitter from its vesicles (3). 5-HT receptors are located on both pre- and postsynaptic membranes. Presynaptically, 5-HT$_{1B}$ (auto)receptors negatively regulate 5-HT release The most common postsynaptic receptors are 5-HT$_{1A-F}$, 5-HT$_{2A/C}$ and 5-HT$_3$ subtypes (4). The hallucinogen lysergic acid diethylamide (LSD) and the anxiolytic buspirone are partial agonists at 5-HT$_{2A}$ and 5-HT$_{1A}$ receptors respectively. After release, 5-HT is taken up into the terminal by the reuptake transporter (5). This is the site of action of many antidepressant drugs, including tricyclic antidepressants (TCAs) and selective serotonin reuptake inhibitors (SSRIs). 5-HT in the terminal is metabolised to 5-hydroxyindoleacetic acid (5-HIAA) by MAO-A (6). This process can be blocked by monoamine oxidase inhibitors (MAOIs), including clorgiline and pargyline.

the brain. Hence, changes in the availability of brain tryptophan will alter brain 5-HT levels.

▪ Tryptophan enters the brain via the large neutral amino acid transporter in competition with other large neutral amino acids.

▪ Administration of balanced mixtures of amino acids without tryptophan reduces plasma tryptophan by promoting protein synthesis. Administration of competing large neutral amino acids such as valine competitively blocks tryptophan transport into the brain. Thus it is possible to lower brain 5-HT either by reducing plasma tryptophan or by 'flooding' the transport carrier with another amino acid. These two methods have been exploited in studies in humans to investigate the function of brain 5-HT.

- 5-HT is stored in vesicles protected from MAO and is released in response to depolarisation of the nerve terminal. 5-HT is mainly metabolised by MAO-A, but MAO-B also plays a role – and this may be greater when MAO-A is blocked.
- The major mechanism for removing 5-HT from the synaptic cleft is reuptake by the 5-HT transporter, which is inhibited by reuptake inhibitors (selective serotonin reuptake inhibitors (SSRIs) and tricyclic antidepressants (TCAs)). There are two well-described polymorphisms of the 5-HTT: the variable number tandem repeat (VNTR) and the serotonin transporter linked promoter polymorphism (5-HTTLPR). Some studies indicate that these may influence the prevalence of depression and/or antidepressant treatment response.
- Amfetamines, such as *p*-chloroamfetamine, fenfluramine and MDMA (Ecstasy) enter 5-HT nerve terminals via the 5-HT transporter, and cause non-impulse-dependent release of 5-HT.
- 5-HT is metabolised intraneuronally by MAO to form 5-hydroxyindoleacetic acid (5-HIAA), which is actively transported across the blood–brain barrier out of the brain.
- 5-HT release at the terminals is subject to inhibitory autoregulation involving 5-HT_{1B} and 5-HT_{1D} receptors.

5-HT receptors (Fig 1.9)

- There are 14 known 5-HT receptors, all of which are G-protein-coupled except the 5-HT_3 subtype, which is a ligand-gated cation channel.
- The 5-HT_1 group (5-HT_{1A}, 5-HT_{1B}, 5-HT_{1D}, 5-HT_{1E}, 5-HT_{1F} are inhibitory and are negatively coupled to adenylate cyclase. 5-HT_{1A} receptors also couple to an ion channel (G-protein-linked inward rectifying potassium channel (GIRK)).
  - The 5-HT_{1A} receptor is found at both somatodendritic and postsynaptic sites. Somatodendritic 5-HT_{1A} receptors in the dorsal and median raphe nuclei are autoreceptors regulating 5-HT neuronal firing. Postsynaptic 5-HT_{1A} receptors are found in various brain regions, including the hippocampus and periaqueductal grey (PAG), where importantly they regulate behaviours such as resilience, impulsivity and restraint of excessive response to stress. The 5-HT_{1A} receptor may be an important target in the action of antidepressants.
  - 5-HT_2 receptors (5-HT_{2A}, 5-HT_{2B}, 5-HT_{2C}) are excitatory and act through the PLC/IP_3 pathway. 5-HT_{2A} receptors are found in the cortex and are associated with sensory perception. The hallucinogen lysergic acid diethylamide (LSD) is a 5-HT_{2A} receptor partial agonist. 5-HT_{2C} receptors when activated reduce food intake and induce anxiety/panic.
- 5-HT_3 receptors are ligand-gated ion channels and are found in high density in the area postrema and nucleus tractus solitarius. 5-HT_3 receptor antagonists (e.g. ondansetron) have their antiemetic actions in this region. 5-HT_3 receptors are also known to regulate DA release in the nucleus accumbens.

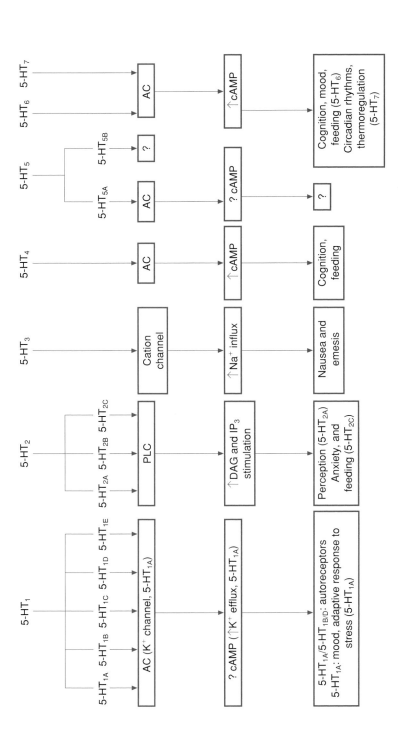

Figure 1.9 Summary diagram of the types of 5-HT receptors, their receptor coupling mechanisms and proposed functions.
AC, adenylate cyclase; cAMP, cyclic adenosine monophosphate; DAG, diacylglycerol; IP$_3$, inositol trisphosphate; PLC, phospholipase C.

The 5-HT_4, 5-HT_6 and 5-HT_7 receptors are positively coupled to AC and are thus excitatory. 5-HT_6 receptor antagonists have been shown in animal studies to modulate memory and attention, while the 5-HT_7 receptor may be important in depression and circadian functions.

Acetylcholine (ACh)

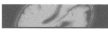

Pathways and functions (Fig 1.3)

- The distribution of ACh in the brain is more diffuse than that of the catecholamines and 5-HT.
- Cholinergic nuclei are located in the basal forebrain and in the pons. The most important nuclei with regard to psychopharmacology are the nucleus basalis of Meynert, which projects to the cortex, and the lateral septum, which sends a projection to the hippocampus (septohippocampal pathway). This latter pathway is disrupted in Alzheimer's disease and is probably associated with the consequent memory dysfunction.
- Cholinergic nuclei in the pons innervate the thalamus.
- Many regions, including the striatum, contain short cholinergic interneurons.

Synthesis and metabolism (Table 1.2, Fig 1.10)

- ACh is synthesised from choline and acetyl coenzyme A (CoA) – a reaction that is catalysed by the enzyme choline acetyltransferase (ChAT).
- ACh is stored in vesicles in the nerve terminals, and is released when the terminal is depolarised.
- Following release, ACh is metabolised by acetylcholine esterase (AChE) to form choline and free acetate. Choline is taken up into the neuron by an active transport system and can then be reused to sythesise ACh.
- Drugs that inhibit AChE are used in the symptomatic treatment of Alzheimer's disease (see Chapter 9).

Cholinergic receptors

- These are subdivided into two classes: nicotinic and muscarinic, with further subdivision within the classes.
- Nicotinic receptors are involved in fast excitatory synaptic transmission, and are directly coupled to cation channels.
  - They are pentameric structures comprising α and β subunits.
  - There are two basic types: muscle (found at the neuromuscular junction) and neuronal (widespread in the central nervous system (CNS)).
  - In the brain, receptors composed of α_4 and β_2 subunits ($\alpha_4\beta_2$) and receptors composed entirely of α_7 subunits (α_7 homomers) are the most common, although $\alpha_3\beta_4$ are also present.

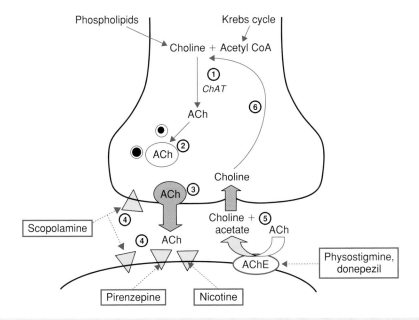

Figure 1.10 Schematic model of a central cholinergic terminal indicating possible sites of drug action. Acetylcholine (ACh) is synthesised from choline and acetyl coenzyme A (CoA) by choline acetyltransferase (ChAT). (1) ACh is stored in vesicles, but there are no clinically effective drugs that act at this site (2). There is some evidence that aminopyridines and phosphatidylserines release ACh and may have limited use in Alzheimer's disease patients (3). Presynaptic muscarinic autoreceptors (4) negatively regulate ACh release. Antagonists at these receptors may have potential in the treatment of Alzheimer's disease, but existing drugs have poor brain penetration and short half-lives. Postsynaptic receptors are of both muscarinic and nicotinic subtypes. In the synaptic cleft, ACh is broken down by acetylcholinesterase (AChE) to form acetate and choline. AChE is a major target for the pharmacotherapy of Alzheimer's disease, but to date AChE inhibitors show only limited efficacy in mild to moderate dementia (5). Choline is transported back into the neuron and recycled (6).

- The different receptor subtypes have different distributions and distinct pharmacology.
- The effects of nicotine on nicotinic receptors on DA neurones in the midbrain are considered to be responsible for the rewarding (and addictive) properties of smoking.
- There are five muscarinic receptors ($M_1, \ldots, M_5$), all found in the brain.
  - They are G-protein-coupled and either activate formation of IP_3 (M_1, M_3, M_5) or inhibit cAMP (M_2, M_4).
  - M_1 receptor agonists and M_2 (autoreceptor) antagonists offer potential targets for the treatment of Alzheimer's disease.

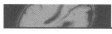 ## γ-Aminobutyric acid (GABA)

Organisation and functions, synthesis and metabolism (Table 1.2)

▦   GABA neurons are widely distributed within the brain, with the highest densities in the basal ganglia, hypothalamus, amygdala and other limbic areas.

▦   GABA is formed by decarboxylation of glutamate catalysed by the enzyme glutamic acid decarboxylase (GAD), which exists in two isoforms (GAD65 and GAD67).

▦   Following release, GABA can either be taken up into the nerve terminals by a specific transport system or enter glial cells where it undergoes mitochondrial metabolism back to glutamate (*GABA shunt*).

▦   The major psychopharmacological interest in GABA is the role of the GABA$_A$ receptor complex in the action of benzodiazepines (BDZs), barbiturates, alcohol and neurosteroids (Fig. 1.11 and see Chapter 6).

GABA receptors

▦   GABA acts on two types of receptor: the GABA$_A$ receptor, which is a ligand-gated ion channel, and the G-protein-linked GABA$_B$ receptor.

▦   GABA$_A$ receptors are composed of five subunits, each of which can occur in multiple isoforms. Usually there are two α, two β, and a single γ subunit. There are six known α isoforms, three β isoforms and two γ isoforms. Receptors of different subunit composition have different pharmacology (Fig 1.11).

▦   The GABA$_A$ receptor (or more properly 'GABA$_A$ receptor complex') is directly coupled to a Cl⁻ ion channel, and its activation results in an influx of Cl⁻ and rapid hyperpolarisation (causing neuronal inhibition).

▦   Barbiturates bind to a site on the GABA$_A$ receptor complex and increase the probability of channel opening in response to GABA, resulting in increased neuronal inhibition. At high concentrations, they can have direct actions in the absence of GABA, and hence cause respiratory depression in overdose.

▦   BDZs bind to a separate site on the GABA$_A$ receptor complex and facilitate the action of GABA, so increasing the frequency of chloride channel opening. Because they require GABA to be present for their action, BDZs are less toxic in overdose than barbiturates.

–   BDZs are agonists at their binding sites, and their actions can be blocked by antagonists (e.g. flumazenil), while inverse agonists at the BDZ site decrease GABA transmission (Fig 1.11).

–   Newer hypnotics such as zopiclone have similar actions to BDZs, but interact with specific subunits of the GABA$_A$ receptor – which may reduce the adverse effects (such as memory loss and dependence).

▦   The GABA$_A$ receptor complex is also modulated by ethanol and neurosteroids, which act at distinct sites.

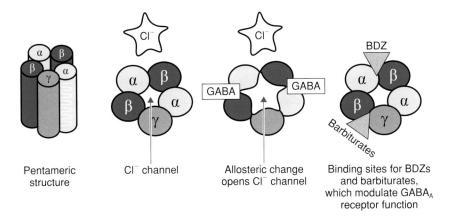

Pentameric structure | Cl⁻ channel | Allosteric change opens Cl⁻ channel | Binding sites for BDZs and barbiturates, which modulate GABAₐ receptor function

Figure 1.11   The γ-aminobutyric acid GABA_A receptor complex is a pentameric structure composed of α_2, β, and (usually) γ subunits arranged to form a central pore. Activation of the GABA_A receptor by GABA or agonists causes a conformational change opening the pore and allowing Cl⁻ ions to flow into the cell causing hyperpolarisation. The GABA_A receptor complex has multiple binding sites. Benzodiazepines (BDZs) are agonists at a site that modulates the ability of GABA to bind to its own site. Agonists at this site facilitate GABA binding whereas inverse agonists reduce it. Barbiturates, neurosteroids and ethanol also modulate GABA_A receptor function. Bicuculline is an antagonist of the GABA_A binding site while muscimol is an agonist at that site. There are multiple forms of each subunit, and receptors composed of the different subunits have different brain distributions and functions. For example, receptors containing α_1 subunits appear to mediate sedation while those containing α_3 subunits mediate anxiolysis. Drugs that can distinguish between receptors with the various subunit isoforms hold promise as selective nonsedating anxiolytics and anticonvulsants.

▪ There are also GABA_B receptors in the brain, at both pre- and postsynaptic sites. These receptors produce slow inhibitory potentials through an increase in K⁺ conductance and inhibit adenylate cyclase. The physiological and behavioural significance of these receptors is not well understood, but they may be important in absence seizures, cognitive performance and the regulation of amine release.

 ## Glutamate

Organisation and functions, synthesis and metabolism (Table 1.2)

▪ Glutamate (a so-called excitatory amino acid) is the major fast-acting excitatory neurotransmitter in the brain.
▪ The cell bodies of glutamatergic neurons are widely distributed in the brain. The pyramidal cells of the cerebral cortex and of the hippocampus are glutamatergic.
▪ Glutamatergic (pyramidal) neurons in the cerebral cortex project to other cortical regions and to subcortical areas. The perforant path from the entorhinal cortex to the hippocampus is also glutamatergic.

■ Glutamate is synthesised from glucose (in the Krebs cycle) or from glutamine. Synthesis takes place in virtually all neurons and glia. Glutamatergic neurons uniquely express a vesicular glutamate transporter that is responsible for the sequestration of glutamate into synaptic vesicles.

■ There are two major reasons for the growing interest in brain glutamate:
   – the link between glutamate (NMDA) receptor activation and long-term potentiation (LTP) in the hippocampus as the physiological substrate of memory
   – the link between excessive glutamate receptor activation and neuro-degeneration caused by loss of intracellular Ca^{2+} homeostasis.

■ There is interest in the role of glutamate transmission in psychosis (schizophrenia) and anxiety. Antagonists at glutamate receptors are as yet of limited clinical use. The dissociative anaesthetic agent ketamine and the psychotomimetic phencyclidine (PCP, Angel Dust) are NMDA receptor antagonists.

Glutamate receptors

■ Glutamate acts on both ligand-gated ion channels (NMDA, α-amino-3-hydroxy-5-methyl-4-isoxazole propionate (AMPA), and kainate receptors) and G-protein-linked or metabotropic receptors (mGluR1–8).

■ AMPA, kainate and NMDA receptors comprise four or more protein subunits. AMPA consists of GluR1–4 (recently renamed GLU_{A1-4}) subunits, kainate of GluR5–7 (GLU_{K5-7}) and KA1 and KA2 (GLU_{K1-2}) subunits, while the NMDA receptor is made of NR1 (GLU_{N1}) subunit(s), together with NR2A–D (GLU_{N2A-D}) and NR3A–B (GLU_{N3A-B}) subunits.

■ AMPA receptors are permeable to Na^+ whilst NMDA receptors are permeable to both Na^+ and Ca^{2+}. The latter receptor is blocked by Mg^{2+} ions.

■ Metabotropic glutamate receptors are divided into three groups: group I (mGluR1, 5) group II (mGluR2, 3), and group III (mGluR4, 6, 7, 8). Drugs acting at mGluRs can influence excitotoxicity and epileptiform activity.

 # References

Further reading

Bear MF, Connors BW, Paradiso MA. Neuroscience Exploring the Brain, 2nd edn. Baltimore: Lippincott, Williams & Wilkins, 2001 (Little on drugs)

Cooper JR, Bloom FE, Roth RH. The Biochemical Basis of Neuropharmacology, 8th edn. Oxford: Oxford University Press, 2003

Hammond C. Cellular and Molecular Neurobiology, 2nd edn. London: Academic Press, 2001 (Neurotransmitter receptor mechanisms)

Leonard BE. Fundamentals of Psychopharmacology, 3rd edn. Chichester: John Wiley, 2003

Rang HP, Dale MM, Ritter JM, Moore PK. Pharmacology, 5th edn. Edinburgh: Churchill Livingstone, 2003 (Pharmacology, not specifically psychopharmacology)

Shiloh R, Stryjer R, Nutt D, Weizman A. Atlas of Psychiatric Pharmacotherapy, 2nd edn. London: Taylor & Francis, 2006

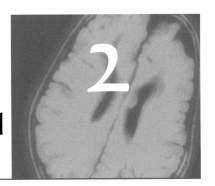

2

Pharmacokinetics and pharmacodynamics

Ian M Anderson

 ## Pharmacokinetics

Basics

- Pharmacokinetics is concerned with the time course and disposition of drugs in the body ('the body's effect on drugs').
- Drugs are intended to act on target organs, but usually have to be given systemically.
- *Bioavailability* (how much of an administered drug reaches its target) is determined by three main factors:
  - absorption
  - distribution
  - elimination (metabolism and/or excretion).
- The *law of mass action* states that 'the rate of a reaction is proportional to the active masses of the reacting substances'. This results in:
- *First-order kinetics* (Figure 2.1), where the rate of absorption or elimination is directly proportional to the amount of drug remaining (for non-reversible reactions). This applies to most psychopharmacological drugs.
- *Zero-order kinetics* (Figure 2.1), where a fixed amount of drug is absorbed or eliminated for each unit of time independent of drug concentrations, because of some other rate-limiting factor. Examples are the metabolism of alcohol and phenytoin (saturation of metabolic enzymes) and absorption of controlled release drugs and depot antipsychotics.

Figure 2.2 shows the hypothetical plasma concentration after drug administration.

- Following drug administration, there is a rise and fall in plasma concentration determined by the processes of absorption, distribution and elimination.
- C_{max} is the maximum plasma concentration achieved.
- $t_{1/2}$ is the time for the plasma concentration to fall by a half (elimination half-life) – in this case by first-order kinetics.
- The *area under the curve* (AUC) after a single dose is proportional to the amount of drug in plasma and allows determination of the fraction of dose absorbed – the bioavailability.

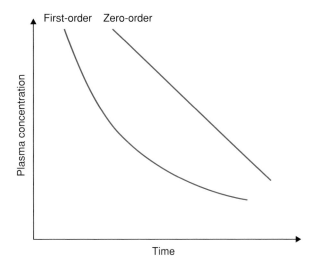

Figure 2.1 In elimination with zero-order kinetics, concentration falls steadily in a straight line, whereas with first-order kinetics, the curve is exponential.

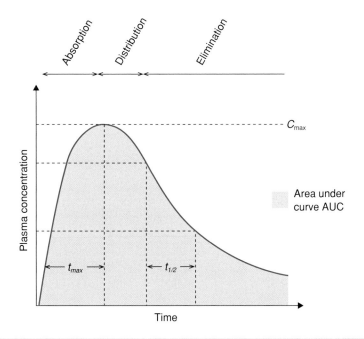

Figure 2.2 Plasma drug concentration in the phases of absorption, distribution and elimination.

Different routes of administration and relevant features are described in Table 2.1.

Absorption

- Absorption is influenced by the route of administration and drug properties.
- Drug delivery systems allow modification of absorption (e.g. enteric coating or delayed-release tablets, depot preparations).
- Liquid preparations (e.g. risperidone, fluoxetine) and oral dispersible tablets (e.g. olanzapine, risperidone, mirtazapine) are aimed at ensuring administration/improving compliance. They generally have minimal effects on absorption.

Table 2.1 Comparison of routes of drug administration

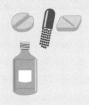 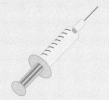 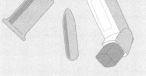

Oral	Parenteral	Other

▪ Most common route, but leads to variable plasma concentration because:
  – Absorption may be erratic
  – Drugs are subject to metabolism by liver (*first-pass effect*)
▪ To be absorbed, drugs must be:
  – Soluble in gastrointestinal fluids
  – Acid-resistant
  – Able to pass across cell membranes, which occurs by passive diffusion and is dependent on lipid solubility
▪ Gastric juice is strongly acid, causing weak acids to be un-ionised and readily absorbed (vice versa for weak alkalis)
	Intravenous
	▪ Most rapid method
	
	Intramuscular
	▪ Absorption occurs over 10–30 minutes
	▪ Rate is dependent on:
	  – Blood flow
	  – Aqueous solubility
	▪ Depot preparations are solutions of drugs in inert oil allowing slow absorption
	
	Other
	▪ Include subcutaneous, intrathecal, etc. (not currently used in psychiatric practice)
		Not generally used in psychiatric practice. Includes:
		▪ Transcutaneous
		▪ Across mucous membranes (e.g. sublingual, rectal)
		▪ Inhalation

Distribution (Fig. 2.3)

▦ During the (re)distribution phase in plasma, the drug is distributed to various tissues in the body, depending on:
  - plasma protein binding
  - tissue perfusion
  - permeability of tissue membranes
  - active transport out of tissues (P-glycoprotein).
▦ Distribution leads to a fall in plasma concentration and is most rapid after intravenous administration.
▦ Distribution can be viewed as the drug achieving equilibrium between different compartments. An approximation is the two-compartment model; central compartment (plasma) and peripheral compartment (tissues).
▦ The apparent *volume of distribution* ($V_d = Q/C_p$) tells us about the characteristics of a drug (V_d = volume of distribution; Q = quantity of drug; C_p = plasma concentration). When V_d is high, this indicates that the drug has high affinity for tissues outside body water, such as brain and fat.
▦ Drugs may be bound to sites where they exert no effect but that influence distribution and elimination:
  - plasma proteins: if highly bound to these, drugs (e.g. many antidepressants, anticonvulsants and warfarin) may displace each other, leading to increased free plasma concentration
  - fat and other sites, which may only release drugs slowly, leading to persistence of drugs in the body (e.g. antipsychotics).

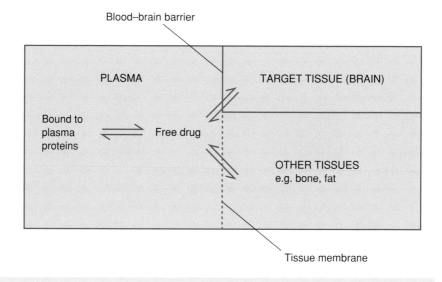

Figure 2.3 Distribution of drug between different body 'compartments'.

- The *blood–brain barrier* is a consequence of the special nature of capillaries in the brain and only allows lipid-soluble molecules into the brain (most psychotropic drugs are lipid-soluble):
  - non-lipid-soluble drugs require special transport systems, which may be active (e.g. L-tryptophan, levodopa) or passive (e.g. lithium)
  - *P-glycoprotein* is an endothelial membrane protein that pumps drugs out of capillary cells by an ATP-dependent process and effectively prevents some drugs getting into the brain (e.g. the opioid loperamide)
  - areas of brain not protected by the blood–brain barrier include the median eminence of the hypothalamus and the vomiting centre.

Elimination (Fig. 2.4)

Metabolism

- Metabolism by the liver is most important, but metabolism may also occur in the plasma, lung and kidney.
- Metabolism may be to active compounds (sometimes called phase I) or to inactive compounds (phase II).
- Non-synthetic reactions:
  - these consist of oxidation, reduction, hydrolysis and demethylation by two main enzyme systems: *cytochrome P450* (CYP450) and *flavin-containing monooxygenase* (FMO)
  - they may produce inactive or active compounds

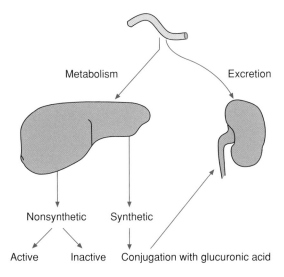

Figure 2.4 Routes of elimination of a drug.

- the CYP450 family of hepatic enzymes are responsible for oxidative metabolism of most psychotropic drugs, with the dominant isoenzyme in drug metabolism being CYP450 3A4 (see Table 2.2 for the most important isoenzymes and examples of their metabolites)
- there is genetic variation in hepatic enzymes affecting rate of metabolism. The most studied is CYP450 2D6. Between 5% and 10% of Caucasians, but only 1–2% of Asians, lack this enzyme and are *poor metabolisers* of the probe drug substrate, dextromethorphan. There are also *extensive metabolisers* of dextromethorphan. In contrast, up to 25% of East Asians are poor metabolisers for CYP450 2C19. Genotyping for some CYP450 isoenzymes (*pharmacogenetics*) is now clinically available, but its utility is still unclear
- *N*-oxygenation by FMO is grouped into five families (1–5). FMO appears to be less important in drug metabolism than CYP450, it is rarely inhibited by compounds and it is implicated less in toxic reactions. Its substrates include clozapine and olanzapine.

▦ Synthetic reactions (conjugation):
- these are usually with glucuronic acid by uridine diphosphate glucuronosyltransferases (UDPGT), of which families 1 and 2 are the most important for glucuronidation of drugs
- they produce inactive, water-soluble compounds.

▦ Factors influencing metabolism:
- there is genetic variation in the activity of CYP450 enzymes (see above)
- drug interactions may lead to inhibition or induction of CYP450 enzymes (resulting in decreased and increased metabolism respectively) (see Table 2.2). Important interactions include:
  - fluoxetine increasing plasma tricyclic antidepressant concentrations
  - fluvoxamine increasing plasma clozapine concentrations
  - carbamazepine decreasing plasma concentration of many drugs (including the contraceptive pill).
- drug interactions may lead to inhibition or induction of glucuronidation. This is the mechanism by which valproate reduces lamotrigine metabolism, leading to increased plasma concentrations
- drugs may compete for the same metabolic pathway (decreasing metabolism of both)
- liver impairment decreases metabolism; liver function may be impaired due to increased age.

Excretion

▦ Excretion by the kidneys is most important, but it may occur through the lungs or in bile, sweat, milk and saliva.
▦ It may be of the active drug or its metabolites:
- ionised and non-lipid-soluble compounds are excreted best
- lithium is the most important drug primarily excreted by the kidneys.
▦ Factors influencing excretion:

Table 2.2 The main cytochrome P450 (CYP450) isoenzymes, with examples of important psychotropic drug substrates, inducers and inhibitors[a]

	CYP450 isoenzymes				
	1A2	**2C9**	**2C19**	**2D6**	**3A3/4**
Substrates	Clozapine	Fluoxetine	Diazepam	Donepezil	Benzodiazepines
	Duloxetine	Phenytoin	Tricyclic	Duloxetine	Ca^{2+} channel
	Haloperidol	Warfarin	anti-	Fluoxetine	blockers
	Olanzapine		depressants	Galantamine	Carbamazepine
	Tricyclic			Mirtazapine	Clozapine
	anti-			Paroxetine	Quetiapine
	depressants			Risperidone	Reboxetine
				Tricyclic	Tricyclic
				anti-	anti-
				depressants	depressants
				Typical	
				antipsychotics	
				Venlafaxine	
Inducers		Phenobarbitone	Carbamazepine		Carbamazepine
					Phenytoin
Inhibitors	Fluvoxamine		Fluvoxamine	Antipsychotics	Fluoxetine
			Fluoxetine	Duloxetine	Nefazodone
				Fluoxetine	
				Paroxetine	

[a]This list is not comprehensive, and it is important to consult a formulary such as the British National Formulary for interactions when prescribing.

- reduction in renal blood flow (nonsteroidal anti-inflammatory drugs, dehydration)
- alterations in reabsorption: urine pH (e.g. alkaline diuresis reduces aspirin reabsorption and increases excretion), low sodium increases lithium reabsorption and decreases excretion
- decreased renal function due to renal impairment, increased age (decreases excretion).

Elimination half-life and steady-state concentration (Fig. 2.5)

- *Steady-state concentration* is achieved after repeated doses lead to an equilibrium between absorption and elimination:
  - this is dependent on dose, time between doses and elimination half-life
  - it is achieved after 4–5 half-lives; doses given at greater intervals than the half-life lead to large fluctuations in plasma concentration

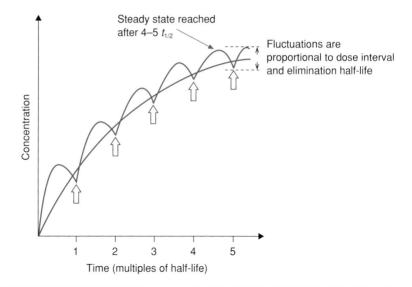

Figure 2.5   Plasma concentration of a drug after repeated administration.

- – delayed-release preparations that slow absorption are an attempt to reduce plasma fluctuations with daily dosing (e.g. venlafaxine, lithium) or to allow long intervals between administrations (e.g. depot antipsychotics)
- Large initial doses (*loading doses*) may be given to achieve therapeutic plasma concentrations more rapidly (e.g. valproate for mania).
- Some drugs have a recognised *therapeutic range* of plasma concentrations (e.g. lithium).
- The *therapeutic index* is the ratio of the minimum plasma drug concentration causing toxic effects to that causing a therapeutic effect. A low therapeutic index (e.g. lithium, phenytoin) usually requires monitoring of plasma/serum concentrations.

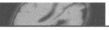 # Pharmacodynamics

Basics

- Pharmacodynamics is the study of the mechanism of drug action ('the effect of drugs on the body').
- Most psychoactive drugs affect the function of specific neurotransmitters either directly or indirectly (see the next section).
- Drugs affecting monoamine neurotransmitters (dopamine (DA), noradrenaline (NA) and serotonin (5-HT)), are important in the treatment of psychotic and affective disorders.
- Drugs acting on amino acid neurotransmitters (γ-aminobutyric acid) (GABA) and glutamate), are important in the treatment of anxiety disorders and epilepsy.

- There is increasing interest in drugs acting on other neurotransmitters (e.g. peptides, nitric oxide).
- Alteration of neurotransmitter function is also commonly responsible for *side-effects* (unwanted or adverse effects).
- Drugs may also act at sites that directly alter neuronal function (e.g. anaesthetics, alcohol).

Sites of drug action on neurotransmitters (Fig. 2.6)

1. *Synthesis* (e.g. L-tryptophan is the precursor of 5-HT, and its administration results in increased 5-HT synthesis).
2. *Storage* (e.g. reserpine depletes NA and DA stores in nerve terminal vesicles).
3. *Release* (e.g. amfetamine releases NA and DA into the synapse.)
4. *Reuptake* (e.g. tricyclic antidepressants (TCAs) inhibit monoamine reuptake into the presynaptic neuron and so increase neurotransmitter concentration in the synapse).
5. *Degradation* (e.g. monoamine oxidase inhibitors (MAOIs) prevent the breakdown of monoamine neurotransmitters).
6. *Receptors* (e.g. antipsychotics antagonise DA receptors).
7. *Other postsynaptic mechanisms* (e.g. lithium inhibits second-messenger function).

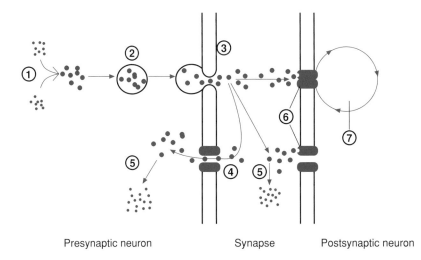

Presynaptic neuron   Synapse   Postsynaptic neuron

Figure 2.6   Sites of drug action on neurotransmitters (for key to numbers, see text).

Agonists

- *Agonists* are drugs that mimic endogenous neurotransmitters.
- Most drugs bind reversibly to receptors, and in the simplest case the response is proportional to the fraction of receptors occupied (*law of mass action*).
- As the concentration of drug increases, the response increases until all the receptors are occupied, giving a *dose–response curve* as shown in Fig. 2.7. When maximum effects are achieved without full receptor occupancy, there are said to be *spare receptors*.
- In Fig. 2.7, the two *full agonists* (A and B) are able to bring about maximum responses; however, A does so at a lower concentration than B because it has a greater *affinity* for the receptor.
- Drug C in Fig. 2.7 has a lower *efficacy* than A and B and does not cause a maximal response even when all receptors are occupied – it is a *partial agonist* (e.g. buspirone, buprenorphine, aripiprazole). Partial agonists can partially antagonise the effect of full agonist (see the next section and Fig. 2.9).
- The *potency* of a drug is determined by:
  - the proportion of the drug reaching the receptor
  - its affinity for the receptor
  - its efficacy.

Antagonists

- *Antagonists* bind to receptors without causing an effect and they block the action of agonists, causing a reduced effect for a given concentration of agonist (a shift to the right of the dose–response curve for the agonist).

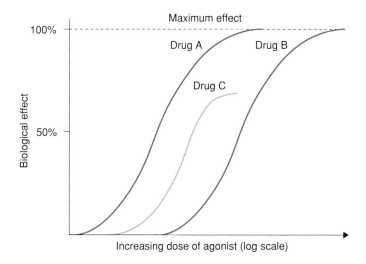

Figure 2.7   Different pattern of responses to agonists (see the text for explanation).

- Most antagonist drugs are *competitive* and are displaced from their binding site by agonists, so that at high doses the agonist can still exert maximum effect (Fig. 2.8a). This competition is influenced by the relative affinity of the agonist and antagonist for the receptor.
- *Noncompetitive antagonists* cannot be displaced by agonists and not only shift the curve to the right but also reduce the maximum effect (Fig. 2.8b). Noncompetitive antagonists may be reversible if the system is restored to normal when the antagonist is removed, or irreversible if restoration of function requires synthesis of new receptors.
- In the presence of a full agonist, increasing concentrations of a partial agonist will antagonise the response until the level of its intrinsic activity is reached (Fig. 2.9). Higher doses of a high-affinity partial agonist therefore 'set' a level

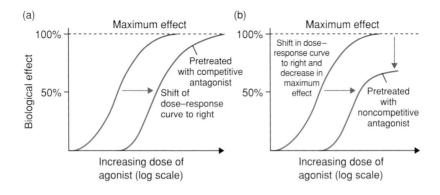

Figure 2.8   Effect of antagonists on the action of agonist drugs (see the text for explanation).

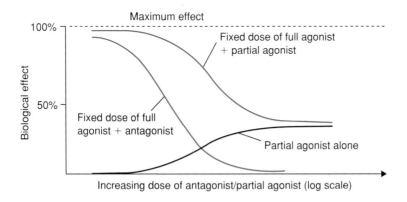

Figure 2.9   Effect of increasing doses of a partial agonist alone and in the presence of a full agonist (see the text for explanation).

of neurotransmission that is independent of the concentration of agonist (e.g. it is proposed that aripiprazole *'stabilises'* DA neurotransmission, avoiding both over- and underactivity, possibly resulting in benefit to both positive and negative symptoms of schizophrenia without causing extrapyramidal side-effects).

Tolerance and sensitisation

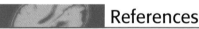 *Tolerance* describes the diminished response to the administration of a drug after repeated exposure. It may be caused by:
  - increased metabolism (e.g. carbamazepine increases the activity of enzymes that metabolise it (*enzyme induction*))
  - reduced receptor sensitivity or number (*downregulation*)
  - activation of a homeostatic mechanism (e.g. in the second-messenger or effector system)
  - behavioural tolerance through learning to cope with the effects.
- *Cross-tolerance* between drugs is the basis for a number of drug interactions (e.g. alcohol with barbiturates; carbamazepine with oral contraceptives).
- *Sensitisation* is the enhancement of drug effects following the repeated administration of the same dose of drug (e.g. stimulants such as amfetamines in animals).

References

Further reading

Cooper JR, Bloom FE, Roth RH. The Biochemical Basis of Neuropharmacology, 8th edn. Oxford: Oxford University Press, 2003

Feldman RS, Meyer JS, Quenzer LF. Principles of Neuropsychopharmacology. Sunderland, MA: Sinauer Associates, 1997

King J (ed). Seminars in Clinical Psychopharmacology, 2nd edn. London: Gaskell, 2004

Schatzberg AF, Nemeroff CB. The American Psychiatric Publishing Textbook of Psychopharmacology, 3rd edn. Arlington, MA: APPI, 2004

Shiloh R, Stryjer R, Nutt D, Weizman A. Atlas of Psychiatric Pharmacotherapy, 2nd edn. London: Taylor & Francis, 2006

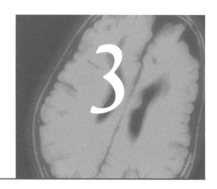

Antipsychotics

Michael J Travis and Ian C Reid

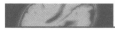 ## History

Like the antidepressants, antipsychotic drugs were discovered by chance.

- *1950s*: Phenothiazines were developed. Chlorpromazine was originally synthesised as an antihistamine/antihelminthic, but was subsequently found to be sedative and antipsychotic. More compounds were synthesised within the same and related classes (e.g. thioxanthines; see Table 3.1). The butyrophenones were created in the late 1950s: haloperidol began life as a candidate analgesic, and was later found to have antipsychotic properties. Further compounds were synthesised in this and other classes (e.g. phenylbutylpiperidine).
- *1970s*: Atypicals were developed (see Table 3.2). They were classified as 'atypical' on the basis of reduced extrapyramidal side-effects in animal models (e.g. thioridazine, sulpiride).
- *1980s*: Clozapine was 'rediscovered', with recognition of its broader efficacy compared with other antipsychotics.
- *1990s*: New-generation atypical antipsychotics were introduced: amisulpride, olanzapine, quetiapine, risperidone, sertindole, ziprasidone.
- *2000s*: First partial dopamine (DA) agonist antipsychotic introduced: aripiprazole.

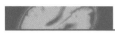 ## The dopamine hypothesis

The DA system (see Chapter 1) is believed to play an important role in the action of antipsychotic drugs.

Key findings

- *1960s*: Antipsychotics were found to increase the turnover of brain DA.
- *1970s*: The greater the DA receptor-binding affinity of an antipsychotic, the greater the clinical potency (Fig. 3.1).

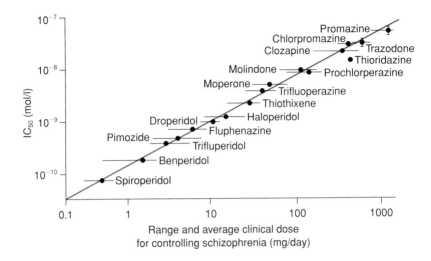

Figure 3.1   Affinity for dopamine receptors and clinical potency. Source: Reprinted with permission from Creese et al. 1976. Copyright © 1976, American Association for the Advancement of Science.

■ *1980s*: α- but not β-flupentixol has greater antipsychotic activity than placebo (only the α isomer is an antagonist at D_2 receptors) (Fig. 3.2).

■ *1990s*: Enhanced amfetamine-induced release of DA in patients with schizophrenia compared with controls, observed using single photon emission computed tomography (SPECT) imaging, implies presynaptic DA system abnormalities in schizophrenia (Fig. 3.3).

■ *Late 1990s*: A series of neurochemical imaging experiments indicates that above approximately 60% of striatal D_2-like receptor occupancy predicts antipsychotic efficacy, while greater than approximately 80% predicts the onset of extrapyramidal side-effects (EPSE) (Fig. 3.4).

Role of dopamine receptor subtypes
(see also Chapter 1)

Although typical and most atypical antipsychotics have many different pharmacological effects, they share the property of blocking the D_2 receptor subtype. However:

■ 20–50% of patients do not respond to D_2 antagonists.

■ Some atypical antipsychotics achieve an antipsychotic effect without high D_2 occupancy.

■ There is no consistent evidence from positron emission tomography (PET) studies or genetic association studies to suggest a constitutional change in D_2 receptors per se in schizophrenia. Minor abnormalities found are probably secondary to regulatory alteration.

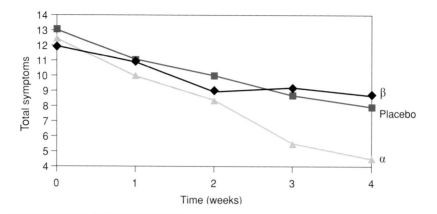

Figure 3.2 Efficacy of α- and β-flupentixol in schizophrenia. The α-isomer caused a greater improvement in symptomatology than placebo, while the β-isomer was without antipsychotic efficacy. Source: Reproduced with permission from Johnstone et al. 1978.

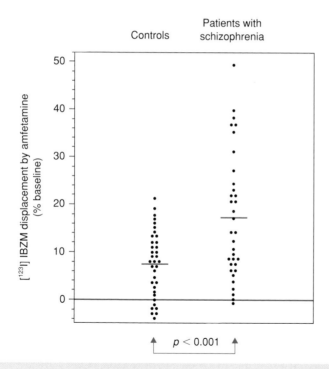

Figure 3.3 Dopamine transmission and schizophrenia. This graph illustrates the effect of amfetamine (0.3 mg/kg) on [^{123}I]IBZM binding in healthy control subjects and untreated patients with schizophrenia. The results indicate that when challenged with amfetamine, patients with schizophrenia release more dopamine than healthy controls. The amount of release is related to the increase in positive symptoms. Source: Reproduced with permission from Laruelle et al. 1996.

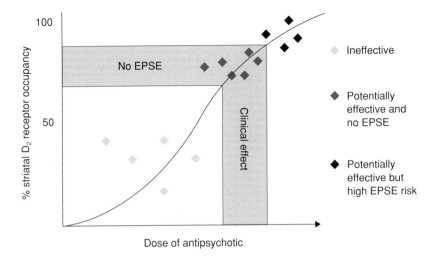

Figure 3.4 D$_2$-like receptor occupancy levels, clinical efficacy and side-effects. D$_2$ receptor occupancy of 60–80% is associated with efficacy with minimal extrapyramidal side-effects (EPSE).

The role of D$_3$ and D$_4$ receptor subtypes is also uncertain:

- Some atypical antipsychotics have a high affinity for D$_3$ and D$_4$ receptors.
- D$_3$ and D$_4$ receptors are distributed in proportionately higher densities in limbic areas.
- Genetic association studies suggest that abnormal D$_3$ variants (but not D$_4$ variants) may occur in excess in patients with schizophrenia.
- Some postmortem studies suggest that D$_3$ and D$_4$ receptor densities may be greater in the schizophrenic brain.
- Some D$_4$ antagonists, however, do not have antipsychotic properties.

Therapeutic actions of antipsychotic drugs

- The chemical classification of older and newer antipsychotics is given in Tables 3.1 and 3.2 and their clinical uses in Table 3.3.
- Given that each of the newer antipsychotics belongs to a different chemical class, attention has turned to delineating their different pharmaceutical properties.
- In the UK, the National Institute for Clinical Excellence (NICE 2002) has given guidance on the use of atypical antipsychotics in schizophrenia, recommending their use as first-line treatment based on their side-effect profile. NICE (2002) has also issued general guidelines for the treatment of schizophrenia.

Table 3.1 Chemical classification of older 'typical' antipsychotics

Chemical class	Drug
Phenothiazine:	
Aliphatic side-chain	Chlorpromazine
Piperidine side-chain	Thioridazine[a]
Piperazine side-chain	Trifluperazine
	Fluphenazine
Thioxanthene	Flupentixol
	Zuclopenthixol
Butyrophenone	Haloperidol
	Droperidol[b]
Diphenylbutylpiperidine	Pimozide
Substituted benzamide	Sulpiride[c]

[a]Use restricted due to ↑QTc.
[b]Withdrawn due to ↑QTc.
[c]Considered by some to be an 'atypical' antipsychotic.

Table 3.2 Chemical classification of newer 'atypical' antipsychotics

Chemical class	Drug
Dibenzodiazepine	Clozapine
Thienobenzodiazepine	Olanzapine
Dibenzothiazepine	Quetiapine
Benzisoxazole	Risperidone
Imidazolidinone	Sertindole
Substituted benzamide	Amisulpride
Quinolinone	Aripiprazole

Table 3.3 Clinical indications for antipsychotics

Psychiatric	Non-psychiatric
Treatment of psychosis	Nausea
Treatment of mania	Anaesthesia (neuroleptanalgesia,
Sedation/ tranquillisation	premedication)
Severe anxiety	Intractable hiccough
? Depression	Terminal illness

- However, there remains some uncertainty about the benefits of atypical antipsychotics in clinical use. A recent large randomised controlled trial (RCT) (CATIE) did not find consistent differences between atypical antipsychotics and perphenazine over 18 months, with 64–82% of patients stopping the assigned drug and equal numbers stopping treatment because of intolerable side-effects.

Sedation and tranquillisation

- Tranquillisation is related to DA receptor-blocking action.
- Sedation is related to the antihistamine action and the α-adrenergic blocking properties (phenothiazines are therefore very sedative).
- See Chapter 9 for the use of antipsychotics in rapid tranquillisation.

Antipsychotic action

The reduction of acute, positive schizophreniform symptoms (i.e. hallucinations, delusions, some aspects of thought disorder, sometimes called 'neuroleptisation') is related to DA receptor-blocking action.

Some relevant clinical findings in the treatment of acute-phase schizophrenia

- In the 1964 National Institutes of Mental Health study, 463 patients with acute schizophrenia were each given a 6-week trial of chlorpromazine, fluphenazine, thioridazine or placebo. Seventy-five percent of the patients improved on antipsychotics, compared with 25% on placebo.
- Antipsychotics alone are as good as antipsychotics plus psychotherapy. Both are better than psychotherapy alone or milieu therapy. Electroconvulsive therapy (ECT) is better than psychotherapy, but not as good as antipsychotics. (Note that ECT is not recommended by NICE for schizophrenia in the UK; see Chapter 4.)
- A meta-analysis of placebo-controlled trials with chlorpromazine showed that it was better than placebo in all 26 studies at doses over 400–500 mg per day.
- An influential study by Kane et al (1988) showed that clozapine was more effective than chlorpromazine (30% vs 4% response) in 268 treatment-resistant patients, with improvement in both positive and negative symptoms.
- The CATIE study randomised 1432 patients with chronic schizophrenia to typical or atypical antipsychotics. Over 18 months, olanzapine was the most effective in terms of the rates of discontinuation; the efficacy of perphenazine was similar to that of quetiapine, risperidone and ziprasidone. Olanzapine was associated with greater weight gain and increases in measures of glucose and lipid metabolism, while perphenazine was associated with more discontinuation for EPSE.

Relapse prevention

Antipsychotics also protect against relapse of positive symptoms.

- When patients stable on depot were transferred to either fluphenazine or placebo for 9 months, 8% of patients on fluphenazine relapsed, compared with 66% on placebo.
- In a review of 66 studies (covering 1958–1993), with follow-up of about 8 months, the relapse rate in the medication-withdrawal groups was 53%, compared with 16% in the maintenance groups.
- In a review of 22 patient cohorts comparing gradual with abrupt discontinuation of medication, abrupt discontinuation resulted in a cumulative relapse rate of about 46% at 6 months and 56% at 24 months; gradual reduction halved the 6-month relapse rate.

 # Adverse effects of antipsychotic drugs

Extrapyramidal side-effects (EPSE)

Motor side-effects are generated by the blockade of DA receptors in the basal ganglia (see Chapter 1). They are now more rarely seen in patients treated with the newer atypical antipsychotics, but may be seen when higher doses are used. There are four main forms (Table 3.4).

Acute dystonia and pseudo-parkinsonism

- These effects are more likely with antipsychotics that have no intrinsic anticholinergic action (e.g. butyrophenones), and are less likely with antipsychotics with intrinsic anticholinergic properties (e.g. phenothiazines). This is because of the reciprocal actions of DA and cholinergic systems in the basal

Table 3.4 Extrapyramidal side-effects of antipsychotics

1. Acute dystonia Oculogyric crisis Torticollis Tongue protrusion Facial grimacing	*3. Akathisia*
	4. Tardive syndromes Dyskinesia Dystonia Akathisia
2. Pseudo-parkinsonism Muscular rigidity Resting tremor Akinesia	

ganglia. These side-effects, by definition, are also less likely with atypical antipsychotics.

- Treatment of EPSE:
  - reduce dose
  - change drug to an atypical antipsychotic
  - introduce anticholinergic medication, e.g. procyclidine or trihexyphenidyl (benzhexol). These drugs should not be co-prescribed with antipsychotics routinely (i.e. in the absence of EPSE), as there is potential for abuse and they may retard antipsychotic effects. Some studies suggest that up to 80% of patients chronically treated with anticholinergics can have the medication withdrawn without adverse effect
  - DA agonists (e.g. bromocriptine) may be used to treat persistent rigidity/akinesia. There is, however, a theoretical risk of aggravation of psychosis symptoms.

Akathisia

- This is a highly unpleasant physical and psychological restlessness.
- The precise cause is unknown and it is difficult to treat:
  - the simplest strategy is dose reduction – anticholinergics do not appear to confer benefit
  - diazepam and β-blockers may be helpful.

Tardive syndromes

- These are serious, disfiguring and often permanent movement disorders.
- The most common manifestation is tardive dyskinesia (Table 3.5), but dystonia and akathisia may also be present or predominate. It most commonly causes involuntary movement of the mouth or tongue, although any muscle groups may be affected.
- The mechanism by which tardive dyskinesia occurs is poorly understood. Most theories focus on the disruption of D_1/D_2 receptor stimulation balance by antipsychotics, but a significant incidence of dyskinesia has also been observed in untreated schizophrenic patients.
- The disorder affects about 40–50% of long-term-treated patients, usually coming on after months to years of treatment (hence 'tardive'), but cases have been reported after a single episode of exposure to an antipsychotic. The incidence is highest in the first few years of treatment, with men and women equally affected.
- The risk of tardive dyskinesia increases with age, and it may occur in normal ageing without antipsychotic exposure. The emergence of tardive dyskinesia is not predicted by the dose of antipsychotic used, or by whether anticholinergic medication has been employed.
- Treatment of tardive dyskinesia:
  - if possible, the antipsychotic (and any associated anticholinergic) medication should be gradually withdrawn or reduced: an initial exacerbation of the dyskinesia can be expected

Table 3.5 Signs of tardive dyskinesia

Ocular muscles	*Neck*
Blinking	Retrocollis
Blepharospasm	Torticollis

Facial	*Trunk*
Spasms	Shoulder shrugging
Tics	Pelvis rotation or thrusting
Grimaces	Diaphragmatic jerks
	Rocking

Oral	Forced retroflexion
Pouting	
Sucking	*Limbs*
Lip smacking	Finger movements
Pursing	Wrist torsion and flexion
	Arm writhing or ballismus
Masticatory	Ankle torsion and flexion
Chewing	Foot tapping
Lateral movements	Toe movements

Lingual	*Others*
Tongue protrusion	Generalised rigidity
'Fly-catching' tongue	
Writhing movements	

Pharyngeal
Palatal movements
Swallowing
Abnormal sounds

- consider clozapine as an alternative antipsychotic
- consider benzodiazepines (e.g. clonazepam)
- consider tetrabenazine (a vesicular DA depleter)
- there are open trials of many drugs (e.g. vitamin E), but controlled data are lacking
- neurosurgery (pallidotomy) may be helpful in extreme cases
- up to approximately 55% of patients may show recovery within a year with antipsychotic reduction or switch to clozapine.

Neuroleptic malignant syndrome (NMS)

- This relatively rare (0.5–1% of patients) but severe syndrome is characterised by:

- muscular rigidity
- decreased conscious level
- hyperthermia
- labile blood pressure
- increased creatine kinase.
- The disorder evolves rapidly over 24–72 hours, and lasts for 10–14 days if untreated. Between 5–20% of patients on oral medication and up to 30% of patients on depot formulations who develop the full syndrome will die from the condition if untreated. The usual cause of death is renal failure secondary to rhabdomyolysis.

Treatment of neuroleptic malignant syndrome

- The syndrome represents a serious medical emergency.
    - antipsychotic drugs must be withdrawn immediately
    - dantrolene may be used to reduce muscle spasm
    - the DA agonist bromocriptine may be employed to reverse anti-dopaminergic effects
    - ECT, which activates DA systems, has also been used
    - intensive care facilities may be required.
- If it is necessary to use antipsychotic medication after recovery, a 2-week interval should be observed and a structurally dissimilar antipsychotic gradually introduced with careful monitoring.

Diabetes/metabolic syndrome

- Concern has recently arisen about a link between antipsychotics, especially 'atypical', and diabetes/metabolic syndrome (abdominal obesity, dyslipidaemia, atypical antipsychotics, hypertension, insulin resistance or glucose intolerance, and prothrombotic and proinflammatory states).
- The independent risk due to the drugs themselves is difficult to determine:
    - there is an increased risk of diabetes in schizophrenia itself
    - patients often have unhealthy lifestyles
    - weight gain is common (especially with clozapine and olanzapine)
    - research evidence is conflicting and the difference between drugs is unclear, but clozapine and olanzapine may be the most likely to cause glucose dysregulation.
- When prescribing antipsychotics (especially 'atypicals') screening for diabetes should be considered and active management of its risk factors (e.g. weight gain) should be undertaken.

Cardio/cerebrovascular events

Cardiac conduction effects

- Sudden cardiac death associated with antipsychotic use has long been recognised, but the degree of causality has been debated.
- Recent focus has been on prolongation of the QT interval (usually reported as QTc – corrected for heart rate):
  - epidemiological and ECG studies suggest that antipsychotics differ in their effects on the QT interval and their link with sudden death
  - a likely mechanism is differential blockade by antipsychotics of the delayed rectifier K^+ channel (I_{Kr}) in the myocardium, encoded for by the human ether-a-go-go (HERG) gene
  - these findings have led to a reduction in the maximium recommended dose of haloperidol, restrictions on the use of thioridazine and sertindole with monitoring requirements, and the withdrawal of droperidol (see also Chapter 11)
  - assessment of QTc and cardiovascular status should be considered, especially if higher-risk or high-dose antipsychotics are prescribed.

Stroke

- An increased risk of cerebrovascular events has been reported in patients with dementia treated with risperidone and olanzapine, but this may also apply to other antipsychotics (see also Chapter 8).

Other effects of antipsychotics

See Table 3.6.

Table 3.6   Other possible (non-extrapyramidal) effects of antipsychotics

Anticholinergic	***Hepatotoxicity***
Dry mouth	Chronically raised liver enzymes
Constipation	
Blurred vision	***Weight gain***
	Especially clozapine, olanzapine,
Anti-adrenergic	chlorpromazine
Postural hypotension	
	Blood dyscrasias
Cardiotoxicity	Well known with clozapine, but shared by all
Slowing of cardiac conduction time	antipsychotics to a lesser extent
(increased QTc), leading to sudden	
death (especially thioridazine, pimozide)	***Photosensitivity***
Possibility of causing myocarditis has	Especially chlorpromazine; use sun block
been raised	
	Venous thromboembolism
	Especially low-potency typical antipsychotics
	and clozapine

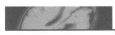 ## Atypical antipsychotics

- The problem of EPSE with 'typical' antipsychotics and the increased efficacy of clozapine compared with other antipsychotics has encouraged the search for 'atypical' clozapine-like drugs without its drawbacks.
- The distinction between 'typical' and 'atypical' is not clear, and some prefer the terms 'older' and 'newer' or 'first-generation' and 'second-generation'.
- However, the differences between drugs means that it is more meaningful to consider drugs individually.

Definitions of atypicality

- A number of factors have been proposed as involved in defining atypicality:
    - greater efficacy for positive symptoms than older antipsychotics
    - greater efficacy for negative symptoms than older antipsychotics
    - lower tendency to cause EPSE than older antipsychotics
    - failure to increase serum prolactin.
- However, the most parsimonious definitions are related to a decreased tendency to cause EPSE:
    - *preclinically*: an effective antipsychotic that does not produce catalepsy in rats; or
    - *clinically*: a drug with wide therapeutic ratio for antipsychotic effects and EPSE such that EPSE are not seen at clinically effective doses.

The wide therapeutic range can be conceptualised as two doses: a lower dose and an upper dose. The lower dose is that at which, in a group of patients, 50% will achieve some clinical benefit – this is the minimum effective dose. The upper dose of this range is the dose of an antipsychotic medication at which 50% of the group of patients will experience some form of mild EPSE. The older, 'typical', antipsychotics generally had a very narrow dose range, roughly equating to 6–7 mg of haloperidol equivalents. The newer, 'atypical', antipsychotics generally have a much wider range. This allows the prescribing physician to predict a dose of one of the newer medications that is likely to be effective but unlikely to cause EPSE. This was much more difficult with the older medications.

Mechanisms of atypicality

Atypical antipsychotics vary in their pharmacological properties. It is likely that a number of mechanisms confer different aspects of atypical status:

- Reduced EPSE:
  - lower D_2 antagonism
  - high 5-HT_2 : D_2 binding ratio
  - limbic selective D_2 antagonism
  - 'loose binding' to dopamine D_2-like receptors
  - D_2 partial agonism
  - cholinergic M_1 antagonism (note that high levels of M_1 antagonism may exacerbate psychosis).
- Reduced hyperprolactinaemia:
  - lower D_2 antagonism
  - D_2 partial agonism.
- Increased efficacy against positive symptoms. Proposed mechanisms include:
  - differential D_1 binding
  - high 5-HT_2 : D_2 ratio
  - high D_4 binding
  - other relative binding/activity ratios.
- Increased efficacy against negative symptoms. Proposed mechanisms include:
  - pre- versus postsynaptic D_2 antagonism
  - 5-HT_2 antagonism
  - D_2 partial agonism
  - absence of EPSE may simulate a beneficial effect on negative symptoms.

Clozapine represents the prototypical atypical antipsychotic, illustrating the features described above:

- low incidence of EPSE
- does not stimulate prolactin secretion
- effective in treatment-resistant cases
- improves negative as well as positive symptoms
- receptor binding affinity profile: $H_1 > M_1 = \alpha_1 > 5\text{-}HT_2 > D_2 = D_1 = \alpha_2$
- relatively low affinity for the D_2 receptor
- D_2 limbic selectivity.

Distribution of pharmacological mechanisms among atypical drugs

- High affinity for cholinergic M_1 receptors: thioridazine, clozapine.
- Lower affinity for striatal D_2 receptors: clozapine, quetiapine, olanzapine.
- Higher affinity for 5-HT_{2A} receptors than for striatal D_2 receptors: risperidone, sertindole, ziprasidone, olanzapine, clozapine, quetiapine.
- Higher affinity for limbic D_2 and D_2-like receptors than for striatal D_2 receptors: clozapine, sertindole, amisulpride, quetiapine, risperidone (any limbic selectivity is lost at higher doses for all, except possibly clozapine).
- 'Loose binding' to striatal D_2-like receptors: clozapine, quetiapine(?), risperidone(?), sertindole(?), olanzapine(?) (but this may be a pharmacokinetic rather than a pharmacodynamic effect).
- D_2 partial agonism: aripiprazole.

Individual atypical antipsychotics (listed alphabetically)

- Currently, amisulpride, aripiprazole, olanzapine, quetiapine, risperidone, sertindole (with restrictions) and zotepine are licensed in the UK.

Amisulpride

Pharmacology

- Selective and equipotent antagonism for D_2 and D_3 receptors.
- Limbic-selective.
- Negligible affinity for other receptors.

Efficacy

- As efficacious as haloperidol for acute and chronic schizophrenia.
- Optimum dose 400–800 mg/day.
- At 50–300 mg, effective for patients with mainly negative symptoms.

Side-effects

- Low rate of EPSE (similar to placebo) at lower doses.
- Less weight gain than with risperidone or olanzapine.
- Dose-dependent EPSE and prolactinaemia at higher doses.

Aripiprazole

Pharmacology

- D_2 partial agonist.
- Partial agonist at 5-HT_{1A} receptors.
- High-affinity antagonist at 5-HT_{2A} receptors.
- Low/moderate affinity antagonist at H_1 and α_1 receptors.
- No anticholinergic effect.

Efficacy

- As effective as haloperidol and olanzapine for acute and chronic schizophrenia.
- Optimum dose 10–15 mg/day (maximum 30 mg).
- Effective in acute treatment of mania.

Side-effects

- Low rate of EPSE (similar to placebo) at all doses (initial akathisia can occur in the first 2 weeks of treatment).

- Does not increase plasma prolactin levels (and may decrease them).
- Less weight gain than with olanzapine.

Olanzapine

Pharmacology

- Related to clozapine.
- Receptor antagonism: $5\text{-HT}_2 = H_1 = M_1 > D_2 > \alpha_1 > D_1$.
- Some D_2 limbic selectivity.
- Available in short-acting injection form.

Efficacy

- As effective as haloperidol for positive symptoms of schizophrenia.
- Some evidence of better efficacy against negative symptoms of schizophrenia.
- Better than risperidone for mood symptoms.
- Effective in acute treatment of mania and maintenance treatment of bipolar disorder.

Side-effects

- EPSE similar to placebo at clinical doses.
- Sedation.
- Weight gain.
- Dizziness.
- Dry mouth.
- Constipation.
- Less increase in prolactin than with haloperidol or risperidone.
- Possible glucose dysregulation.

Quetiapine

Pharmacology

- Receptor antagonism: $H_1 > \alpha_1 > 5\text{-HT}_2 > \alpha_2 > D_2$.
- D_2 limbic selectivity.

Efficacy

- As effective as haloperidol and chlorpromazine for schizophrenia.
- Possible efficacy for negative symptoms.
- Effective in acute treatment of mania and continuation treatment and is effective in bipolar depression.

Side-effects

- EPSE equivalent to placebo.
- No increase in prolactin.
- Sedation.
- Dizziness.
- Constipation.
- Less frequent: dry mouth, weight gain.

Risperidone

Pharmacology

- Receptor antagonism: $5\text{-}HT_2 > D_2 = \alpha_1 = \alpha_2$.
- Little histamine H_1 affinity.
- Minimal D_1, $5\text{-}HT_1$ affinity.
- D_2 limbic-selective only at lower doses.
- Available in long-acting injectable form.

Efficacy

- There have been at least 11 multicentre double-blind trials in schizophrenia.
- Possible bell-shaped dose–response curve.
- Uncertain if effective for negative symptoms.
- Effective in acute treatment of mania and continuation treatment in bipolar disorder.

Side-effects

- Markedly less pseudoparkinsonism than with typical antipsychotics at lower doses, but dystonias and akathisia can occur.
- Tachycardia.
- Some weight gain.
- Fewer treatment dropouts than with typical antipsychotics in RCTs.

Sertindole

This was withdrawn due to concerns about increases in QTc. There was a limited reintroduction in 2002 in Europe under strict monitoring.

Pharmacology

- D_2, $5\text{-}HT_2$ and α_1 antagonist.
- D_2 limbic selectivity.

Efficacy

- Effective against positive and negative symptoms of schizophrenia.

Side-effects

- EPSE equivalent to placebo.
- Minimal short-term increase in prolactin.
- Increase in QTc: needs ECG monitoring.
- Nasal congestion, decreased ejaculatory volume, postural hypotension and dry mouth.
- Occasionally raised liver enzymes.

Ziprasidone

This is licensed in the USA and parts of Europe, but not in the UK.

Pharmacology

- Receptor antagonism: $5\text{-HT}_{2A} > D_2 > 5\text{-HT}_{1A} > \alpha_1 > H_1$.
- Possible limbic selective D_2 antagonism.
- No anticholinergic effect.
- Weak 5-HT and NA reuptake inhibition.

Efficacy

- Perhaps slightly more effective than haloperidol.
- Possible efficacy for negative symptoms of schizophrenia.
- Possible efficacy for depressive symptoms in schizophrenia.
- Effective in acute treatment of mania.

Side-effects

- EPSE equivalent to placebo.
- No appreciable weight gain.
- No appreciable cholinergic side-effects.
- Insomnia, pharyngitis, rash and tremor more common than with placebo.
- Concerns over tendency to increase QTc.
- Appears to reduce prolactin relative to placebo.
- Headache, nausea and insomnia most common side-effects (but occur in <10% of patients).

Zotepine

Pharmacology

- High affinity for D_1 and D_2 receptors, also 5-HT_2, 5-HT_6 and 5-HT_7 receptors.
- Inhibits NA reuptake.

Efficacy

▪ Effective against positive and negative symptoms of schizophrenia, but controlled trial data limited.

Side-effects

▪ EPSE less than typical antipsychotics.
▪ Seizures at higher doses (> 300 mg).
▪ Weight gain.
▪ Sedation.
▪ Constipation, asthenia, dry mouth, akathisia.
▪ Raised hepatic enzymes.

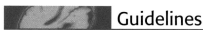 # Guidelines

National Institute for Clinical Excellence Technology Appraisal No. 43. Guidance on the use of newer (atypical) antipsychotic drugs for the treatment of schizophrenia, 2002. http://www.nice.org.uk/page.aspx?o=appraisals.completed
National Institute for Clinical Excellence Clinical Guideline 1. Schizophrenia: Core interventions in the treatment and management of schizophrenia in primary and secondary care, 2002. http://www.nice.org.uk/page.aspx?o=guidelines.completed

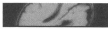 # References

Key references

Bollini P, Pampallona S, Orza MJ et al. Antipsychotic drugs: Is more worse? A meta-analysis of the published randomised controlled trials. Psychol Med 1994; 24:307–16
Creese I, Burt DR, Snyder SH. Dopamine receptor binding predicts clinical and pharmacological potencies of antischizophrenic drugs. Science 1976; 192:481–3
Cunningham-Owens DG. Adverse effects of antipsychotic agents. Do newer agents offer advantages? Drugs 1996; 51:895–930.
Geddes J, Freemantle N, Harrison P, Bebbington P. Atypical antipsychotics in the treatment of schizophrenia: systematic overview and meta-regression analysis. BMJ 2000; 321:1371–6
Hirsch S, Gaind R, Rohde PD et al. Outpatient maintenance of chronic schizophrenia patients with long-acting fluphenazine: double-blind placebo trial. BMJ 1973; i:633–7
Johnstone E, Crow TJ, Frith CD et al. Mechanism of the antipsychotic effect in the treatment of schizophrenia. Lancet 1978; i:848–51
Johnstone EC, Crow TJ, Frith CD, Owens DG. The Northwick Park 'functional' psychosis study: diagnosis and treatment response. Lancet 1988; ii:119–25
Kane J, Honigfeld G, Singer J, Meltzer H. Clozapine for the treatment-resistant schizophrenic: a double-blind comparison with chlorpromazine. Arch Gen Psychiatry 1988; 45:789–96
Lieberman JA, Stroup TS, McEvoy JP et al. Clinical Antipsychotic Trials of Intervention Effectiveness (CATIE) Investigators. Effectiveness of antipsychotic drugs in patients with chronic schizophrenia. N Engl J Med 2005 353:1209–23

Viguera AC, Baldessarini RJ, Hegarty JD et al. Clinical risk following abrupt and gradual withdrawal of maintenance neuroleptic treatment. Arch Gen Psychiatry 1997; 54:49–55

Wyatt RJ. Neuroleptics and the natural course of schizophrenia. Schizophr Bull 1991; 17:325–51

Further reading

Busatto GF, Kerwin RW. Perspectives on the role of serotonergic mechanisms in the pharmacology of schizophrenia. J Psychopharmacol 1997; 11:3–12

Carpenter WT, Jr. Maintenence therapy of persons with schizophrenia. J Clin Psychiatry 1996; 57(Suppl 9):10–18 (This whole supplement is good)

Davis JM, Andriukaitis S. The natural course of schizophrenia and effective maintenance treatment. J Clin Psychopharmacol 1986; 6(Suppl 1):2–10

Gilbert PL, Harris J, McAdams LA, Jeste DV. Neuroleptic withdrawal in schizophrenic patients. Arch Gen Psychiatry 1995; 52:173–88

Haddad P, Dursun S, Deakin B. Adverse Syndromes and Psychiatric Drugs: A Clinical Guide. Oxford: Oxford University Press, 2004

Hegarty JD, Baldessarini RJ, Tohen M et al. One hundred years of schizophrenia: meta-analysis of the outcome literature. Am J Psychiatry 1994; 151:1409–16

Kuperberg G, Kerwin R, Murray R. Developments in the pharmacological treatment of schizophrenia. Expert Opin Invest Drugs 2002; 11:1335–41

Laruelle M, Abi-Dargham A, van Dick et al. Single photon emission computerized tomography imaging of amphetamine-induced dopamine release in drug-free schizophrenic subjects. Proc Natl Acad Sci USA 1996; 93:9235–40

Laruelle M, Abi-Dargham A, Gil R et al. Increased dopamine transmission in schizophrenia: relationship to illness phases. Biol Psychiatry 1999; 46:56–72

Malhotra AK, Litman RE, Pickar D. Adverse effects of antipsychotics drugs. Drug Safety 1993; 9:429–36

McGurk SR, Meltzer HY. The effects of atypical antipsychotic drugs on cognitive functioning in schizophrenia. Schizophr Res 1999; 25:233–55

Seeman P, Guan HC, van Tol HH. Dopamine D4 receptor elevated in schizophrenia. Nature 1993; 365:441–5

Seeman P. Atypical antipsychotics: mechanism of action. Can J Psychiatry 2002; 47:27–38

Staddon S, Arranz MJ, Mancama D et al. Clinical applications of pharmacogenetics in psychiatry. Psychopharmacology 2002; 162:18–23.

Stahl S. Essential Psychopharmacology: Neuroscientific Basis and Practical Implications, 2nd edn. Cambridge: Cambridge University Press, 2000

Taylor D. Low-dose typical antipsychotics – a brief evaluation. Psychiatr Bull 2000; 24:465–8

Taylor D, Paton C, Kerwin RW. The South London and Maudsley NHS Trust 2006 Prescribing Guidelines, 8th edn. London: Taylor & Francis, 2006

Travis MJ. Schizophrenia and other psychotic disorders: therapeutic armamentarium. In: D'haenen H, den Boer JA, Willner P (eds). Biological Psychiatry. Chichester: John Wiley, 2003: 685–700

Travis MJ, Burns T, Dursun S, et al. Aripiprazole in schizophrenia: consensus guidelines. Int J Clin Pract 2005; 59:485–95

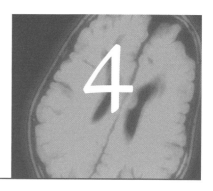

Antidepressants and ECT

Ian C Reid

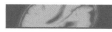

History

The first effective antidepressant agents of the modern era were discovered by chance in the late 1950s:

- Iproniazid (monoamine oxidase inhibitor, MAOI): originally developed as an antitubercular drug.
- Imipramine (tricyclic antidepressant, TCA): originally developed as a chlorpromazine analogue (1957).
- MAOIs and TCAs have the common property of interacting with monoamine systems (dopamine (DA), noradrenaline (NA) and serotonin (5-HT)).

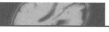

The monoamine hypothesis of depression

The monoamine hypothesis was originally proposed in the 1960s based on the actions of drugs (reserpine was observed to cause depression and antidepressants to relieve depression).

- Schildkraut proposed that catecholamines (NA, DA) were functionally deficient in depression and elevated in activity in mania.
- Ashcroft proposed that indoleamines (5-HT) were functionally deficient in depression. This led to the development of 5-HT-selective drugs in the 1970s, resulting in the selective serotonin reuptake inhibitors (SSRIs).
- The hypothesis has been much modified over succeeding decades, with the focus moving from neurotransmitter turnover, through receptor regulation, to intracellular changes.
- A current formulation proposes that a common mechanism of antidepressant action is to increase 5-HT neurotransmission by altering receptor sensitivity.
- For example, chronic 5-HT reuptake blockade with SSRIs results in down-regulation of 5-HT_{1A} receptors on the cell bodies of serotonergic neurons in the brainstem, thus disabling negative feedback, restoring cell firing rate and resulting in increased synaptic 5-HT (Fig. 4.1).

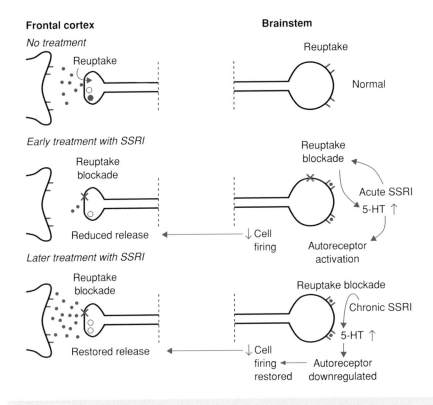

Figure 4.1 Current serotonin (5-HT) hypothesis of how antidepressant drugs work. SSRI, selective serotonin reuptake inhibitor.

- The hypothesis does not satisfactorily explain the similarity in efficacy of very different agents acting differentially on monoamine systems.
- Furthermore, evidence for primary monoamine disturbance in depressed subjects is limited and somewhat inconsistent.

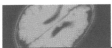 # Evidence for the role of monoamines in the aetiology of major depression

The action of antidepressants on monoamine neurotransmission does not by itself mean that these systems are abnormal in depression. The main evidence is summarised below:

Serotonin (5-HT)

- Reduced 5-HT metabolites in the cerebrospinal fluid of sufferers, and in brain tissue postmortem.

- Increased platelet/brain 5-HT$_2$ receptors.
- Downregulation/reduced numbers of postsynaptic 5-HT$_{1A}$ receptors (neuro-endocrine studies: decreased prolactin response to tryptophan infusion and reduced buspirone-induced hypothermia; positron emission tomography (PET) studies showing reduced brain 5-HT$_{1A}$ receptor binding).
- Relapse of depression induced by tryptophan depletion in SSRI-treated and drug-free recovered depressed patients.

Noradrenaline (NA)

- Reduced levels of the NA metabolite MHPG in the urine of depressed subjects.
- Possible postsynaptic α_2 downregulation (neuroendocrine studies: reduced growth hormone response to the α_2-agonist clonidine and to insulin-induced hypoglycaemia).
- Decreased responses to β-receptor agonists in depression.
- Relapse of depression induced by α-methylparatyrosine (NA synthesis inhibitor) in patients treated with NA reuptake inhibitors.

Dopamine (DA)

- Increased D$_2$ receptor numbers in some PET studies of depressed patients.
- Mood-elevating effects of DA-releasing psychostimulants.
- Possible antipsychotic-induced depression (high dose: postsynaptic DA receptor blockade).
- Possible antipsychotic antidepressant activity (low dose: presynaptic DA autoreceptor blockade leading to increased DA release).
- Preclinical studies consistently implicate DA systems in neural basis of reward (related to anhedonia).

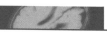 ## The role of the HPA axis

Abnormalities in the regulation of the hypothalamic–pituitary–adrenal (HPA) axis are implicated in the aetiology of depressive disorder, although they are not specific to depressive disorder nor are they demonstrable in every case.

- Many depressed patients exhibit elevated cortisol levels and an insensitivity to dexamethasone-induced cortisol suppression (the dexamethasome suppression test).
- Complex interactions between 5-HT and corticosteroid systems in the central nervous system (CNS) are only now beginning to be understood, and may account for some of the relationships between the effects of stress, mood dysregulation and cognitive dysfunction encountered in depressive disorder.

- The toxic effects of cortisol dysregulation may account for the evidence of degenerative changes (e.g. reduced hippocampal volume) seen in the brain in depressive disorder.
- Adverse early experience – physical, emotional, or sexual abuse – may alter HPA axis function in a lasting way, conferring vulnerability to depression and stress-related disorders in adulthood.
- Recent trials suggest that glucocorticoid receptor antagonists (e.g. mifepristone), may be effective treatments in severe depressive disorder. Hormones that regulate the HPA axis, such as corticotropin-releasing factor (CRF), and other agents active at the various glucocorticoid and mineralocorticoid receptors in the brain, are attracting interest as potential targets for developing future antidepressants.

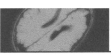 # The neurotrophic and neuroplasticity hypotheses

- Recent research indicates that in chronic severe depressive disorders, alterations in brain structure may occur, particularly frontal and temporal cortical atrophy, possibly mediated by corticosteroid abnormalities.
- Intriguingly, antidepressant agents (including electroconvulsive stimulation, ECS) have common cellular effects leading to enhanced expression of neuroprotective proteins that bolster neuronal survival and regulate synaptic connectivity:
  - in rats, antidepressant drugs and ECS promote enhanced cell production in the dentate gyrus of the hippocampus. These effects may act to reverse the proposed toxic effects of HPA axis abnormalities (Fig. 4.2)
  - preliminary studies in some stress-related disorders, such as post-traumatic stress disorder, suggest that antidepressant drugs can reverse volumetric abnormalities in limbic system structures, such as the hippocampus.

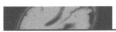 # Antidepressant drugs

Most antidepressants have acute effects on monoamine neurotransmission (Fig. 4.3).

Tricyclic antidepressants (TCAs)

Neurochemical effects: spectrum of activity

- 5-HT reuptake inhibition.
- NA reuptake inhibition.
- Tertiary amines generally more potent at blocking 5-HT uptake.

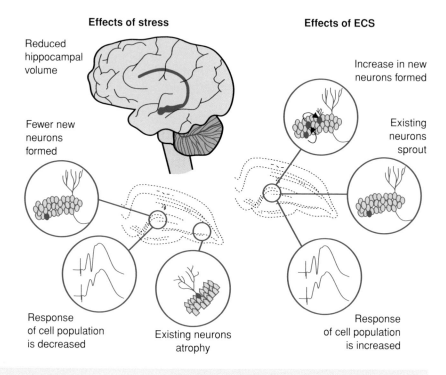

Effects of stress

Reduced hippocampal volume

Fewer new neurons formed

Response of cell population is decreased

Existing neurons atrophy

Effects of ECS

Increase in new neurons formed

Existing neurons sprout

Response of cell population is increased

Figure 4.2 Reciprocal effects of stress and electroconvulsive stimulation (ECS) on neurons. (Courtesy of Dr CA Stewart, University of Dundee.)

- Secondary amines more potent at blocking NA.
- Anticholinergic effects.
- Antihistaminergic effects.

Pharmacokinetics

- Rapidly absorbed, widely distributed.
- Genetic variation in liver metabolism.
- Tertiary amines metabolised to secondary amines, e.g. amitriptyline to nortriptyline; imipramine to desmethylimipramine.
- Comparative pharmacology of TCAs is shown in Table 4.1.

Efficacy

- Acute treatment of episode of depression: 55–70% response rate, 30–50% remission rate, 10–20-day delay in significant improvement (note that there is increasing evidence that antidepressant effects can be detected in the first week).

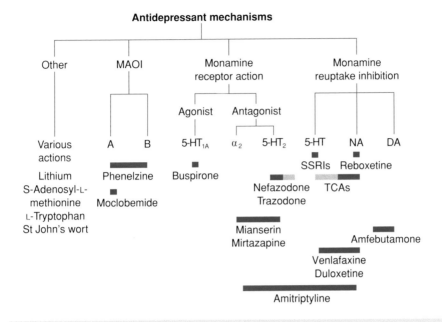

Figure 4.3   Acute pharmacology of some antidepressants. MAOI, monoamine oxidase inhibitor; 5-HT, serotonin; NA, noradrenaline; DA, dopamine; SSRI, selective serotonin reuptake inhibitor; TCA, tricyclic antidepressant.

Table 4.1   Selective comparative pharmacology of tricyclic antidepressants (TCAs)

	$t_{1/2}$ (h)[a]	NA reuptake inhibition	5-HT reuptake inhibition	Anticholinergic	Sedation
Amitriptyline	16 (36)	++	+++	+++	+++
Imipramine	16 (24)	++	+++	++	++
Clomipramine	18 (36)	+	+++	++	+
Nortriptyline	36	+++	+	++	+
Dosulepin (dothiepin)	20 (40)	+	+	++	++
Lofepramine	5 (24)	+++	+	+	+

$t_{1/2}$, half-life; NA, noradrenaline; 5-HT, serotonin.
[a]$t_{1/2}$ of active metabolite in parentheses.

- Effective in relapse prevention.
- Although evidence is inconclusive, probably need adequate dose (125–150 mg imipramine or equivalent) – requires dose titration (inconvenient for doctor and patient).

- Useful in adults, agitation, retardation, severe depression (may be more effective in severe depression in inpatients compared with SSRIs).
- Less useful in the elderly, psychotic, physically ill, those with a history of bipolar disorder and the suicidal.

Side-effects

- *Anticholinergic*: dry mouth, constipation, urinary retention, visual accommodation problems, glaucoma.
- *Antihistaminergic*: sedation, weight gain.
- *α-Noradrenergic blockade*: postural hypotension, sedation.
- *5-HT₂ blockade*: weight gain (especially amitriptyline).
- *Cardiotoxic*: QT prolongation, ST elevation, AV block, membrane stabilisation, arrhythmias.
- *Neurotoxic*: delirium, movement disorders, convulsions.
- *Discontinuation syndrome* (see also SSRIs below): general somatic symptoms, insomnia, vivid dreams, gastrointestinal symptoms, mood symptoms (including anxiety, agitation), rarely psychosis.
- *Manic switch in bipolar patients*.

Contraindications

- Heart block.
- Hypomania or mania.
- Recent myocardial infarction.

Interactions

Useful interactions (with caution)

- SSRIs, lithium, L-tryptophan.

Problematic interactions

- MAOIs (especially clomipramine with tranylcypromine).
- Antiepileptics (barbiturates decrease TCA levels).
- Cimetidine increases TCA levels.
- Warfarin action potentiated.
- Alcohol potentiates TCA sedation.

Selective serotonin reuptake inhibitors (SSRIs)

Increasingly, SSRIs are the first-line treatment for depression.

Neurochemistry

All share the property of relatively selective 5-HT reuptake blockade, but are structurally distinct, and most have some degree of other actions on different neurotransmitter systems, some of which may be as yet undocumented.

Pharmacokinetics

- Rapidly absorbed.
- Hepatic metabolism.
- Some have active metabolites (Table 4.2).
- Variation in cytochrome P450 (CYP450) inhibition and potential for drug interactions (Table 4.2).
- Low concentrations in breast milk (fluoxetine highest).
- Withdrawal effects possible with short-half-life drugs (paroxetine greatest, fluoxetine least).

Efficacy

- Acute treatment of episode of depression: 55–70% response rate, 30–50% remission rate.

Table 4.2 Selective comparative pharmacology of selective serotonin reuptake inhibitors (SSRIs)

	Active metabolite	$t_{1/2}$ (h)[a]	CYP450 inhibition
Citalopram	−	36	−
Escitalopram (S-enantiomer of citalopram	−	36	−
Fluoxetine	+++	72 (200)	+++ (2D6, 3A4, 2C19)
Fluvoxamine	−	15	++ (1A2, 2C19)
Paroxetine	−	20	+++ (2D6, 2C9)
Sertraline	+	25 (66)	+ (2D6)

$t_{1/2}$, half-life; CYP450, cytochrome P450.
[a]$t_{1/2}$ of active metabolite in parentheses.

- 10–20-day delay in significant clinical response (note that there is increasing evidence that antidepressant effects can be detected in the first week).
- Effective in relapse prevention.
- Little evidence for dose-response in usual dose range: less need for dose titration.
- Useful in the elderly, depression with anxiety/obsessive–compulsive disorder (OCD), suicidal patients (safer in overdose than tricyclics).
- There is recent evidence that escitalopram may be more effective, or have an earlier onset of action, than citalopram and have equal efficacy to venlafaxine. This is attributed to escitalopram (S-enantiomer of citalopram) binding to both the reuptake site and an allosteric site causing conformational change in the 5-HT transporter and enhancing reuptake blockade. The R-enantiomer blocks this effect. This is not seen with other SSRIs. These are mostly company data, so claims need independent verification.

Side-effects

- Nausea/vomiting (activation of postsynaptic 5-HT$_3$ receptors).
- Agitation.
- Akathisia.
- Parkinsonism (uncommon).
- Sedation/dizziness (10–20%).
- Convulsions (rare).
- Sexual dysfunction common in males and females (possibly activation of post-synaptic 5-HT$_2$ receptors); appears most prominent with paroxetine, possibly least with fluvoxamine.
- Controversial: increased risk of suicidality, which may be due to agitation/akathisia (see also Chapter 10):
    - in the UK, an expert group was set up in 2003 by the Medicines and Healthcare Products Regulatory Authority (MHRA) to investigate this possible side-effect. They concluded that a modest increase in the risk of suicidal thoughts and self-harm for SSRIs compared with placebo could not be ruled out. This may be particularly apparent in younger patients
    - the same group commented on the use of SSRIs in children and young adults (see Chapter 10)
    - more recent epidemiological studies suggest that suicidality is greatest in the month prior to treatment (and is often a reason for initiating treatment), and begins to fall once treatment has been initiated
    - the implication is that early and frequent monitoring of suicide risk is prudent.
- Recent cohort studies have suggested that paroxetine exposure in the first trimester of pregnancy may increase the risk of ventricular septal defect, cleft-lip/palate and pyloric stenosis. The risk is small, and uncertainty remains as to the causal role of paroxetine.
- Discontinuation syndrome related to half-life (especially paroxetine, rare with fluoxetine) (see below).

Interactions

Useful interactions (with caution)

- TCAs, lithium, L-tryptophan (but may also cause problematic interaction with all).

Problematic interactions (including serotonin syndrome with other serotonergic drugs)

- MAOIs (toxicity).
- L-tryptophan.
- For fluvoxamine (due to CYP450 1A2 inhibition): caffeine, clozapine, theophylline.
- For fluoxetine and paroxetine (due to CYP450 2D6 and 3A3/4 inhibition): antipsychotics, opiates, TCAs.
- St John's wort (serotonin syndrome).

Serotonin syndrome

- Acute toxic syndrome due to increased 5-HT activity (can be confused with neuroleptic malignant syndrome (NMS); see Chapter 3).
- Symptoms:
  - confusion
  - myoclonic jerks, hyperreflexia
  - pyrexia, sweating, autonomic instability (usually less than in NMS)
  - gastrointestinal symptoms
  - mood change, mania.
- Management:
  - stop the offending drug/s: in milder cases especially, symptoms can resolve quickly
  - supportive measures.

SSRI discontinuation syndrome

- Symptoms (usually beginning within 3–5 days of stopping SSRI):
  - sensory abnormalities (including electric shock-like sensations)
  - dysequilibrium (dizziness, etc.)
  - insomnia, increased dreams
  - general somatic symptoms (headache, lethargy, etc.)
  - gastrointestinal symptoms
  - mood change (depression, anxiety/agitation, rarely mania)
  - psychosis (rarely).
- Management:
  - education and reassurance: usually mild and self-limiting over 1–2 weeks
  - if more severe, restart SSRI and taper more slowly; or
  - switch to/start fluoxetine, then withdraw drug.

Monoamine oxidase inhibitors (MAOIs)

Neurochemistry

- Inhibition of MAO enzymes A and B.
- MAO present in periphery, especially the gut, as well as the CNS.
- MAO-A metabolises NA, 5-HT, DA and tyramine.
- MAO-B metabolises DA, tyramine and phenylethylamine.
- MAOIs increase the storage and release of 5-HT and NA.
- Traditional MAOIs (phenelzine, tranylcypromine) and some relatively selective MAO-B inhibitors (e.g. selegiline): irreversible inhibition.
- Selegiline transdermal patches (EMSAM®) licensed in 2006 in the USA for the treatment of depression. This reduces hepatic and digestive tract drug exposure, preserves MAO-A metabolism of dietry tyramine and reduces risk of hypertensive reactions.
- Moclobemide: reversible inhibitor of MAO-A (RIMA) – potential for interaction with indirect sympathomimetics greatly reduced as drug is displaced from enzyme.

Pharmacokinetics

- Rapid absorption.
- Toxic levels can occur in slow acetylators.
- Half-life is not as important as the time taken to replace stores of MAO after irreversible blockade (2 weeks).

Efficacy

Traditional MAOIs are third-line treatment, but retain important place in therapy. Useful in:

- Severe depression, especially with lethargy and poor motivation.
- Treatment resistance: may also be combined with lithium and/or L-tryptophan.
- Atypical depression – now defined as depression with mood reactivity, excessive sleeping and weight gain, sensitivity to rejection as a personality trait (DSM-IV) (older definitions included phobic anxiety).
- anxiety disorders (see Chapter 6).

Side-effects

- Postural hypotension.
- Restlessness, insomnia.
- Peripheral oedema – beware ascites/pleural effusion.
- Nausea, dizziness, sexual difficulties, sweating, tremor.

Interactions

- Hypertensive reaction (see below). Moclobemide has low potential for this interaction because of its selectivity for MAO-A and reversibility; selegiline's reduced potential for this reaction lies in its selectivity for MAO-B at low doses and relative preservation of gut MAO-A when given transdermally.
- Other antidepressants: excitement and hyperpyrexia; combination with SSRIs or serotonergic TCA can cause the serotonin syndrome (see above).
- Pethidine: respiratory depression, coma.
- Alcohol, barbiturates: CNS depression.
- Insulin: impaired blood glucose control.

Hypertensive reaction

- Causes:
    - tyramine-containing foods (dietary tyramine is normally inactivated in the gut by MAO): e.g. cheese, yeast extracts, hung game, some alcoholic drinks, broad bean pods, pickled herring
    - indirect sympathomimetic drugs such as phenylephrine (e.g. non-prescription cold remedies).
- Symptoms:
    - flushing
    - headache
    - increased blood pressure
    - rarely cerebrovascular accident.
- Management:
    - prevention: education, food warning leaflets
    - treatment of hypertensive crisis: α-adrenergic blockade with phentolamine or chlorpromazine.

Contraindications

- Cardiovascular disease.
- Cerebrovascular disease.
- Children.
- Epilepsy.
- Hepatic disease.
- Phaeochromocytoma.
- Hyperthyroidism (tranylcypromine).

Notes on other antidepressants

Phenylpiperazines (e.g. trazodone, nefazodone)

- Relatively weak 5-HT reuptake inhibition.
- 5-HT_2 antagonist properties, which may have antidepressant and anxiolytic properties, as well as reducing the impact of 5-HT reuptake on sexual function.

▓ Relatively safe in overdose.
▓ Trazodone is somewhat sedative; can rarely cause priapism.
▓ Nefazodone was withdrawn from the European market in 2003 due to hepatotoxicity; its use is subject to monitoring of hepatic function in the USA.

Noradrenaline reuptake inhibitors (NARIs)
(e.g. reboxetine)

▓ Relatively specific reuptake inhibitor of NA; may have alerting properties.
▓ Side-effects: insomnia, postural hypotension and anticholinergic-like side-effects probably due to functional interaction between sympathetic and parasympathetic nervous systems.

Serotonin and noradrenaline reuptake inhibitors (SNRIs)

Also known as 'dual action' reuptake inhibitors: e.g. venlafaxine, milnacipran (available in France and Japan) and duloxetine.

Venlafaxine

▓ Selective 5-HT and NA reuptake inhibitor (a 'clean' tricyclic?).
▓ NA reuptake inhibition only evident at higher doses.
▓ May have enhanced efficacy in severe depressive disorder.
▓ Blood pressure needs to be monitored when dose exceeds 200 mg daily.
▓ Recent concerns about cardiac toxicity and toxicity in overdose has led to a reassessment of safety evidence in the UK. Current UK guidance is as follows:
  – specialist supervision is required for initiation of venlafaxine in severely depressed and hospitalised patients who require daily doses of 300mg and above
  – venlafaxine is contraindicated in patients with a high risk of serious cardiac ventricular arrhythmia and uncontrolled hypertension.
▓ Care should be taken in assessing suicidality, as with SSRIs (and indeed all antidepressants).
▓ Can cause significant discontinuation symptoms (see SSRI discontinuation syndrome above).

Duloxetine

▓ 5-HT and NA reuptake inhibitor with weak inhibition of DA reuptake.
▓ Trial data suggest there may be a positive effect on painful physical symptoms in depression.
▓ Concerns have recently been raised in the USA about the possibility of causing liver damage or exacerbating pre-existing liver disease.
▓ The drug should not be used with alcohol, and could prove hazardous for patients who abuse alcohol.

Dopamine reuptake inhibitors

The only currently available DA reuptake inhibitor is amfebutamone (bupropion), which may also inhibit NA reuptake. It is unrelated in structure to other anti-depressants. It is licensed in the USA for depression, but not in the UK (where it is licensed as an adjunct for smoking cessation; see Chapter 7).

- Has been used in combination with SSRIs in the USA for treatment-resistant depression.
- It appears to have anticraving properties and can cause weight loss.
- Side-effects include dry mouth, insomnia, anxiety, gastrointestinal disturbance, sweating and hypertension, and at higher doses it may cause seizures (it is contraindicated if there is a history of epilepsy or an eating disorder where an increased risk of seizures has also been seen).

L-Tryptophan

- Precursor of 5-HT.
- Weak antidepressant, adjunct for MAOIs and TCAs.
- Some sedation; watch for eosinophilia myalgia syndrome, myoclonus and serotonin syndrome.
- Was available only on a named-patient basis in the UK due to concerns about eosinophilia myalgia syndrome, but this restriction was lifted in 2005.

α_2-Adrenoceptor antagonists (e.g. mirtazapine, mianserin)

Mirtazapine

- Also known as a noradrenaline- and serotonin-specific antidepressant (NaSSa).
- $5\text{-}HT_2$, $5\text{-}HT_3$, antihistaminergic and α_2-antagonist.
- Relatively sedative antidepressant (antihistaminergic effects), which may be less at higher doses (possibly due to NA stimulation).
- Activates NA neurons by blocking the negative feedback of NA on presynaptic α_2-adrenoceptors.
- Increased noradrenergic activity stimulates 5-HT neuron activity in the brain-stem (via α_1-adrenoceptors), while blockade of α_2-adrenoceptors on 5-HT terminals in the cortex enhances 5-HT release.

Mianserin

- Similar pharmacology to mirtazapine but also antagonises α_1-adrenoceptors, so preventing NA stimulation of 5-HT neurones and reducing postsynaptic NA effects.
- Associated with blood dyscrasias making blood count monitoring necessary.

Other putative antidepressants

▦ Some drugs used as mood stabilisers (see Chapter 5) also have antidepressant properties (lithium in unipolar and probably bipolar depression, lamotrigine in bipolar depression), with a lack of evidence for others, even though they are commonly used as first-line treatment in bipolar depression (valproate, carbamazepine).

▦ Atypical antipsychotics such as olanzapine and quetiapine may have anti-depressant properties in bipolar depression. Low-dose amisulpride is licensed for dysthymic disorders in some countries (e.g. France).

▦ Agomelatine, a melatonin receptor agonist and 5-HT_{2C} antagonist is likely to be licensed for depression in the near future.

▦ Investigational drugs include CRF antagonists (especially psychotic depression) and neurokinin-1 (NK1) antagonists.

▦ St John's wort shows inconsistent evidence for short-term efficacy in mild–moderate depression.

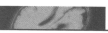 # Using antidepressants effectively

▦ Dose (150 mg imipramine or equivalent) and duration of treatment (at least 6 months post remission) appear to be necessary in attaining stable remission of an acute episode.

▦ Even more important is effective prophylaxis, as depressive episodes are likely to be recurrent – the estimated 3-year relapse rate following adequate treatment is 80% for placebo versus 20% for 150 mg imipramine. Note that 'maintenance dose' is an obsolete concept: the dose that gets you better keeps you better!

▦ Antidepressant use in primary care requires special consideration: there is evidence that antidepressants may be both overprescribed (given to patients with mild disorder who are unlikely to benefit) and underprescribed (following failure to detect illness, or given in insufficient doses for inadequate periods of time).

▦ Meta-analyses suggest that SSRIs may be better tolerated in primary care patients, and because dose titration is less frequently necessary than with TCAs, SSRIs are more likely to be prescribed at therapeutic doses.

▦ A British Association for Psychopharmacology (BAP) evidence-based guideline on the treatment of depressive disorders is available. In the UK, the National Institute for Clinical Excellence (NICE) clinical guideline on the management of depression (2004) emphasises a 'stepped care' model, managing increasing severity of depressive disorder in steps through a range of primary and secondary care settings. Good clinical practice standards of monitoring and patient information are given. NICE guidance in brief:

  – *Mild depression* (primary care, steps 1–2). May be self-limiting, simple psychological therapies, direction to exercise or guided self-help treatment if required. Antidepressant drugs are not routinely recommended.

  – *Moderate to severe depression* (primary care, step 3). Routinely treat initially with an SSRI. Consider psychological therapies (e.g.

cognitive–behavioural therapy (CBT) or interpersonal therapy (IPT)) as alternative or additional treatment. Reserve TCAs, venlafaxine, MAOIs and drug combination treatments for secondary care or specialist settings. Revision of venlaflaxine's licence in 2006 suggests this limitation now only refers to daily doses of 300 mg and above.

- *Treatment-resistant, recurrent, atypical depression or patients at risk (e.g. suicidality)* (specialist practitioners, step 4). Options include combined specific psychological therapies and antidepressant drugs, lithium augmentation, or combination antidepressants (e.g. SSRI and mirtazapine). For patients with recurrent depression resulting in frequent episodes or functional impairment, continuation of treatment for 2 years is recommended.
- *Severe depression, suicide risk or severe self-neglect* (inpatient treatment, step 5). Therapy combinations are as step 4, and patient may require ECT.

- In choosing antidepressant agents, consider:
  - previous response and tolerance, and patient preference
  - side-effect profile in relation to patient characteristics/concerns and need for prophylaxis
  - age and physical health
  - suicidality
  - concordance issues
  - past history of elevated mood: TCAs and venlafaxine may cause manic switch or promote 'rapid cycling' in bipolar disorder
  - possibly symptom profile (e.g. atypical symptoms may respond best to SSRI or MAOI).

Treatment-resistant depression

- Some 20–40% of patients will fail to respond to adequate doses of adequate duration of an antidepressant (usually 6–8 weeks' treatment). In patients who do not respond *at all* to medication after 4 weeks, it is unlikely that the antidepressant will subsequently prove effective. An important exception is elderly patients, who may require longer trials.
- Treatment-resistant depression has varying definitions, but usually refers to a failure to respond to trials of two antidepressants at an adequate dose, given for an adequate period of time (>4 weeks).
- Common strategies following treatment failure include:
  - increasing the dose of the antidepressant drug
  - switching to another drug, often from an alternative class (although even within a class, antidepressants may be chemically very different)
  - adding lithium or triiodothyronine as augmenting agents
  - combining agents (e.g. tricyclic and SSRI; venlafaxine and mirtazapine)
  - electroconvulsive therapy (ECT).
- The 'evidence base' is limited in this situation. With augmentation therapies, the most robust evidence favours the use of lithium, but this may simply reflect the limited research evidence. In any case, it is important to:

- – reconsider the diagnosis
- – appraise concordance with treatment
- – review physical status
- – be systematic in treatment trials.

▦ Careful recording of the history of treatments and their outcomes and adverse events is crucial. Although beyond the scope of this chapter, consideration of specific psychological therapies, such as CBT, is essential.

▦ There are further options:
  - – experimental strategies being investigated include the addition of atypical antipsychotics, the use of modafinil (an antinarcoleptic agent), antiglucocorticoids, and newer physical treatments such as vagus nerve stimulation, transcranial magnetic stimulation and deep brain stimulation. Although promising, their efficacy remains uncertain
  - – very rarely, in extreme cases, neurosurgical approaches, such as anterior cingulotomy, have been used successfully.

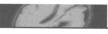Electroconvulsive therapy (ECT)

Although not a psychopharmacological treatment, ECT is considered briefly here because of evidence for similar effects to antidepressant drugs and its place alongside antidepressants in the treatment of severe depression.

History

▦ ECT has its roots in the mistaken idea that schizophrenia and epilepsy are antithetical conditions.

▦ Convulsions were first induced chemically.

▦ Later (in the 1930s), Cerletti and Binet developed the safer electrical induction of seizures. Initially, 'unmodified' ECT was used (i.e. without muscle relaxant).

▦ Now, general anaesthesia and muscle relaxation are employed to reduce the risk of fracture during seizure activity.

▦ Large open trials in the 1960s and blinded, randomised placebo-controlled trials in the 1970s and 1980s demonstrated the efficacy of ECT in depressive disorder.

▦ It remains one of the most controversial treatments in medicine, with a poor 'media' image.

▦ The use of ECT is decreasing. This may be due in part to more systematic and effective drugs and the use of psychological treatment for depressive disorder. However, factors such as adverse public opinion, reduced accessibility because of less frequent inpatient treatment, and loss of professional confidence and experience also appear important. It is uncertain to what degree depressed patients are being denied an effective treatment.

Mode of action

- The mode of action of ECT, like chemical antidepressant therapy, is poorly understood.
- Similar effects on monoamine systems, as occur with chemical antidepressants, have been described; DA systems may be particularly affected.
- Perhaps counterintuitively, there is evidence that electroconvulsive stimulation has neuroprotective effects and stimulates neurogenesis in preclinical models.
- ECT is a potent anticonvulsant, and may share properties with some mood-stabilizing agents effective in affective disorder.
- There is no evidence that ECT causes brain damage.

Indications

- Evidence for efficacy is strongest in depressed patients with psychosis and psychomotor retardation. ECT tends to be reserved for situations where:
  - alternative treatments have failed
  - a rapid response is necessary in the face of intense suicidality
  - there is dangerous self-neglect
  - there are intractable psychotic depressive states.
- NICE guidance in the UK (2003) considered the use of ECT in depression, mania, schizophrenia and catatonia, and recommended the following:
  - its use should be restricted to the short-term and rapid relief of severe depression, mania or catatonia in patients who have failed to respond to other treatments
  - it should not be used in schizophrenia or for maintenance treatment.

Procedure

- The aim of ECT is to induce safely an adequate generalised tonic–clonic seizure.
- Electroencephalographic (EEG) monitoring is now recommended routinely.
- In assessing seizure adequacy, the previous guideline of a minimum 15-second motor seizure and/or a 25-second EEG seizure is no longer deemed applicable with the widespread use of propofol as an anaesthetic agent (associated with shorter seizure durations). Important factors appear to be using an adequate suprathreshold stimulus and achieving high-amplitude synchronous EEG seizure activity. These need to be judged in the context of clinical progress.
- The electrical stimulus is applied via two electrodes placed either bitemporally (bilateral ECT) or across one side of the head (unilateral ECT, to the nondominant hemisphere to minimise cognitive side-effects).
- The dose is measured in units of charge (amps × seconds), and the amount of charge required to induce a seizure may vary 40-fold across individuals, depending on the characteristics of the equipment used.
- Square-wave (brief-pulse) stimuli require less energy to provoke a seizure than sine waves. Increasingly narrower pulses are being given in an attempt to reduce energy and side-effects while maintaining efficacy.

- Given that the intensity of side-effects induced (see below) may vary with the overall electrical energy administered, many authorities advocate stimulus dosing to determine optimal parameters for individual patients.
- Some studies suggest that high-dose unilateral ECT may be as effective as bilateral ECT but is accompanied by less cognitive dysfunction. Bifrontal electrode placement may also reduce cognitive side-effects while maintaining efficacy.
- In general, with ECT, several treatments are required to achieve good outcomes, spaced by 2 or 3 days (i.e. two or three times per week). The median number of treatments given in recent audits in Scotland, England and Wales was six.
- There is considerable variation in the standards of ECT administration, and the Royal College of Psychiatrists in the UK in 2003 set up an ECT accreditation service (ECTAS) to improve practice in England. Scottish practice has been monitored since 1997 and is consistently of a high standard.

Clinical uses

Common

- Depressive disorder not responsive to antidepressants or where rapid response is necessary.
- Treatment-resistant mania.

Less common

- Schizophrenia: ECT may be useful in achieving symptom control in treatment-resistant schizophrenia to permit the use of clozapine (but note that this is not recommended by NICE).

Uncommon

- Catatonia/stupor.
- OCD.
- Movement disorders (e.g. Parkinson's disease).
- Neuroleptic malignant syndrome.

The last three indications were not included in the NICE remit.

Outcome/efficacy

- ECT appears to be extremely effective in depressive disorder, with a response rate greater than that of drug or psychological treatment at 60–80%. A recent meta-analysis confirmed these findings, but the trial base was of limited quality. Patients receiving ECT represent a specific population, generally more severe and 'treatment-resistant' than those receiving other treatments.
- Efficacy and cognitive side-effects appear related to the dose of current applied.

- A direct comparison of matched patients (with random allocation) has not been made with contemporary antidepressant or psychological care.
- Relapse rates are high (especially in treatment-resistant patients), with up to 50% of patients relapsing within the year following treatment.
- Continuation/maintenance ECT appears effective in depressed patients who relapse after successful treatment with ECT, but RCT evidence is lacking. An RCT of continuation ECT (unpublished at the time of writing) is reported not to have shown efficacy in relapse prevention, but there appear to be potential methodological confounds. Maintenance ECT in schizophrenia prevented relapse in a single trial.

Side-effects

- The principal physical hazards of ECT lie with those adverse events encountered generally following brief general anaesthesia. It is recommended that senior anaesthetists experienced in the use of ECT conduct sessions.
- Headache and nausea are common, and respond to conventional treatment.

Cognitive impairment

- Acute confusional state: immediately following treatment, patients are typically disorientated. This lasts for about 20 minutes.
- Anterograde amnesia: patients may experience difficulty in learning new material for a couple of months after treatment. This effect is transient, and may be of less significance than the anterograde learning difficulties seen in untreated depressive disorder.
- Retrograde amnesia: many patients report difficulty in recalling memories that were intact prior to treatment. This is usually restricted to events just prior to each treatment, but, less commonly, a significant minority of patients complain of persistent deficits extending back decades, with patchy loss of autobiographical memories. This impairment is difficult to demonstrate using objective neuropsychological tests.
- In general, it is difficult to disentangle the cognitive effects of depression from those induced by ECT. Often, overall cognitive function improves as depression lifts.
- The Royal College of Psychiatrists now recommends consideration of unilateral ECT as the initial treatment because of concerns about cognitive effects.
- Effects on cognitive function are cumulative throughout the course of ECT. Further treatments after symptom relief has been achieved (e.g. in an effort to bolster response) are not generally justified. However, in patients who are known to relapse rapidly if ECT is stopped at the point of improvement, it may be clinically appropriate to continue with a few further treatments.

Cautions and contraindications

Absolute

- Raised intracranial pressure.
- Recent cerebrovascular accident.
- Unstable vascular aneurysm.
- Recent myocardial infarction with unstable rhythm.

Relative

- Pregnancy.
- Retinal detachment.
- Cerebral tumour.
- History of cerebrovascular accident.

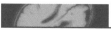 **Guidelines**

Anderson IM, Nutt DJ, Deakin JFW. Evidence-based guidelines for treating depressive disorders with antidepressants: a revision of the 1993 British Association for Psychopharmacology guidelines. J Psychopharmacol 2000; 14:3–20 (available at http://www.bap.org.uk)

National Institute for Clinical Excellence Technology Appraisal Guidance 59. Guidance on the use of electroconvulsive therapy, 2003. http://www.nice.org.uk/page.aspx?o=appraisals.completed

National Institute for Clinical Excellence Clinical Guideline 23. Depression: the management of depression in primary and secondary care, 2004. http://www.nice.org.uk/page.aspx?o=guidelines.completed

Scottish Intercollegiate Guidelines Network National Clinical Guideline 60. Postnatal depression and puerperal psychosis, 2002. http://www.sign.ac.uk/guidelines/published/index.html

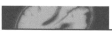 **References**

Key references

Anderson IM, Tomenson BM. The efficacy of selective serotonin re-uptake inhibitors in depression: a meta-analysis of studies against tricyclic antidepressants. J Psychopharmacol 1994; 8:238–49

Charney DS, Menkes DB, Heninger GR. Receptor sensitivity and the mechanism of action of antidepressant treatment: implications for the etiology and therapy of depression. Arch Gen Psychiatry 1981; 38:1160

Cookson J. Side-effects of antidepressants. Br J Psychiatry 1993; 163 (Suppl 20):20–4

Frank E, Kupfer DJ, Perel JM et al. Three-year outcomes for maintenance therapies in recurrent depression. Arch Gen Psychiatry 1990; 47:1093

Geddes J (for the UK ECT review group). Efficacy and safety of electroconvulsive therapy in depressive disorders: a systematic review and meta-analysis. Lancet 2003; 361:799–808

McAllister-Williams RH, Ferrier IN, Young AH. Mood and neuropsychological function in depression: the role of corticosteroids and serotonin. Psychol Med 1998; 28:573–84

Meltzer HY. Serotonergic dysfunction in depression. Br J Psychiatry 1989; 155(Suppl 8):25

Potter WZ, Rudorfer MV, Manji H. The pharmacologic treatment of depression. N Engl J Med 1991; 325:633

Preskorn SH. Pharmacokinetics of antidepressants: Why and how are they relevant to treatment? J Clin Psychiatry 1993; 54(Suppl 9):14–34

Reid IC, Stewart CA. How antidepressants work. Br J Psychiatry 2001; 178:299–303

Stimpson N, Agrawal N, Lewis G. Randomised controlled trials investigating pharmacological and psychological interventions for treatment-refractory depression. Br J Psychiatry 2002; 181:284–94

Further reading

Ashton HA. Brain Function and Psychotropic Drugs. Oxford: Oxford University Press, 1992

Scott AIF (ed). The ECT Handbook, 2nd edn. The Third Report of the Royal College of Psychiatrists' Special Committee on ECT (Council Report CR128). London: Royal College of Psychiatrists, 2005

King J (ed). Seminars in Clinical Psychopharmacology, 2nd edn. London: Gaskell, 2004.

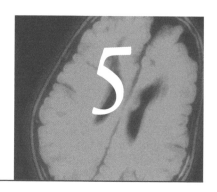

'Mood stabilisers': lithium and anticonvulsants

Allan H Young and Ian C Reid

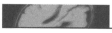 ## What is a mood stabiliser?

- The term 'mood stabiliser' has been applied to lithium and anticonvulsant drugs used to treat bipolar disorder. It is also starting to be applied to some atypical antipsychotics. Its use has become more controversial with developments in anticonvulsant and atypical antipsychotic use in bipolar disorder.
- It refers to the ability of a drug to treat one or both poles of bipolar disorder without causing a switch to the other pole (cf. antidepressants, which can cause a switch to mania), and historically has tended to be used for drugs used in prophylaxis.
- There are, however, problems in its use:
    - should it only be applied to drugs that are effective against both poles?
    - the evidence for efficacy of drugs is often clearer for one pole than the other
    - does it refer to acute or maintenance treatment, or both?
- One suggestion is that drugs can be classified as those that treat from 'Above' (i.e. mania), called type A mood stabilisers, those that treat from 'Below' (i.e. depression), called type B mood stabilisers, and those that are both A and B.
- Some advocate simply referring to a drug's antimanic or antidepressive properties and abandoning the term 'mood stabiliser' altogether.

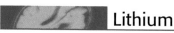 ## Lithium

History

- Lithium is an alkali-metal element that occurs naturally in the mineral petalite. It and its compounds are widely used today in swimming pool filters and batteries for mobile phones and computers.
- The Australian psychiatrist John Cade first proposed the use of lithium salts in the treatment of 'psychotic excitement' in 1949, although its sedative and depressant properties had been known since at least the preceding century.

- Lithium salts were once used extensively as treatment for gout, because lithium urate is particularly soluble and promotes the excretion of urates rather than their deposition in tissue.
- Lithium chloride was briefly used as a sodium salt substitute before its toxicity was properly appreciated.

Mechanism of action

The mode of action of lithium remains only partially understood – there are a range of effects at a number of different levels in the central nervous system (CNS):

- effects on cation transport
- effects on individual neurotransmitters
- effects on intracellular second-messenger systems.

Effects on cation transport

- Increases the activity of Na^+/K^+ adenosine triphosphatase (ATPase) in patients (but, interestingly, not in healthy controls).
- May displace Ca^{2+} and Mg^{2+} ions at a range of sites relevant to neural function, e.g. modulation of Ca^{2+}-dependent activities in the CNS, such as neurotransmitter release.

Monoaminergic neurotransmission

- Decreases DA release from the presynaptic neuron.
- Increases synthesis and release of 5-HT.
- Increases transmission at 5-HT_{1A} receptors.
- Decreases transmission at 5-HT_2 receptors.
- Enhances platelet 5-HT uptake.
- Increases NA uptake into synaptosomes.
- May reduce NA turnover overall in humans.

Cholinergic neurotransmission

- Increases choline levels.
- Enhances cholinesterase inhibitor toxicity.
- Increases growth hormone response to the cholinergic agonist pyridostigmine.

These findings suggest that lithium enhances cholinergic activity in the brain. It is conceivable that these cholinomimetic effects may contribute to antimanic actions, while lithium toxicity resembles atropine poisoning.

Effects on second messengers

Lithium has many interactions with intracellular second-messenger systems and can thus modify signal transduction pathways:

- Inhibits Na^+-induced cyclic adenosine monophosphate (cAMP) activity.
- Limits inositol trisphosphate (IP_3) formation.
- Reduces activity of protein kinases.

The drug can therefore alter the signal induced by multiple neurotransmitter systems, allowing mediation of complex behavioural and physiological responses (see Chapter 1). It is widely believed that these mechanisms account ultimately for the efficacy of the drug.

Neuroprotective effects

- Recent research suggests that lithium has a range of protective effects on neural function and integrity. Bipolar disorder is associated with structural brain changes, and this property may play an important part in the overall efficacy of lithium.
- In animal studies and in isolated human neural cells, lithium has been shown to increase the expression of important neuroprotective proteins.
- Consistent with these effects, lithium appears to increase grey matter volume in patients with bipolar I disorder, to increase the levels of N-acetylaspartate (a putative marker of neuronal viability) in bipolar patients and healthy volunteers, and to enhance neurogenesis in rat hippocampus.
- This evidence suggests that lithium may exert some of its long-term benefits in the treatment of mood disorders via neuroprotective effects and that it may have potential therapeutic properties in neurodegenerative disorders.

Pharmacokinetics

- Rapidly absorbed in the upper gastrointestinal tract.
- Peak serum levels are achieved within 2–3 hours.
- Unbound in serum.
- Excreted unchanged by the kidney at a constant rate proportional to the glomerular filtration rate.
- Steady-state plasma concentration is achieved after 5–7 days.
- Individual lithium preparations have different bioavailability and cannot be substituted dose-for-dose.

Indications

Efficacy in acute mania

- In clinical trials, lithium is effective in 60–80% of acutely ill patients.
- Poorer responses are seen in patients with mixed affective episodes or a rapid cycling pattern.

- Higher levels are required than for prophylaxis.
- Lithium treatment for acute mania was previously considered a first-line strategy in the USA, although in Europe antipsychotic drugs have generally been used as the primary treatment in this situation. This is partly because lithium has little sedative activity of its own.
- Lithium should be used cautiously with antipsychotics because of alleged risks of neurotoxicity when it is combined with high doses of antipsychotic agents.

Bipolar prophylaxis

- Lithium provides effective prophylaxis against mood swings in severe and recurrent bipolar disorder in a proportion of patients. In initial randomised controlled trials, around 80% of patients were reported to benefit. More recent trials, however, suggest poorer results, with 70% of patients relapsing and only 30% having good occupational outcome.
- The decision to commence prophylaxis is based on the frequency and severity of episodes. A traditional rule of thumb has been:
  - after two illnesses within 2 years
  - after three illnesses in 5 years
  - after one severe illness.
- Recent emphasis on the recurrent and progressive nature of bipolar disorder has increasingly led to recommending commencement of prophylaxis after a single manic episode.
- The decision to commence prophylaxis is also governed by likely compliance. Admissions for mania increased after the introduction of lithium:
  - abrupt lithium discontinuation leads to rebound mania (and thus more manic episodes than would have occurred had the drug never been started). A meta-analysis of 19 published studies on lithium discontinuation found that the time to recurrence of affective disorder (mostly mania) was 3 months for 50% of patients
  - as a result, it has been recommended that patients must take the medication for longer than 2 years without discontinuation for benefits to accrue.

Efficacy in routine practice

- Lithium is probably ineffective in approximately 40% of bipolar patients in everyday practice, and there is little doubt that therapeutic use could be improved.
- As noted above, there is an excess recurrence after withdrawal, and short-term use may worsen the course of the illness.
- Despite its long history, lithium use lacks a firm evidence base, and data are particularly limited on its value in bipolar depression.
- There is increasing evidence that lithium may help reduce suicidal ideation and prevent completed suicide.

Unipolar depression treatment and prophylaxis

- Lithium is the best evidenced augmentation strategy for depression that is not responsive to antidepressants (see Chapter 4).
- Lithium is also used in the prophylaxis of recurrent unipolar depressive disorder.
- Controlled trials suggest response rates of 30–40%, and while the strategy is significantly more efficacious than placebo, the magnitude of the effect is small.
- Continuous antidepressant prescription appears more effective than lithium prophylaxis, and its clinical place is as an adjunct to antidepressants in this situation.

Predicting response to lithium

See Table 5.1.

Using lithium

Initiating therapy

Prior to commencing lithium therapy:

- It is important to establish the degree of affective morbidity, both to clarify the indication for therapy and as a reference baseline against which outcome may be judged.
- Because of the danger of rebound mania following discontinuation, the need for prolonged treatment (at least 2 years) should be discussed.

Relevant investigations include:

- Renal function (serum creatinine; full creatinine clearance is usually only needed if there are concerns about renal function).
- Thyroid function.
- ECG (especially if there are cardiac concerns).

Table 5.1   Predictors of response to lithium

Predictors of good response	Predictors of poor response
Greater adherence to treatment	Rapid-cycling bipolar illness
'Pure' form of bipolar illness	Paranoid features
Endogenous/melancholic unipolar illness	Substance abuse
Family history of bipolar illness	Poor psychosocial support
Mania followed by depression	Depression followed by mania
Previous good response to treatment	

- Weight.
- Pregnancy test for females in the years of reproductive potential.

Dosing

- A sensible starting dose is 600–800 mg at night for otherwise healthy individuals.
- Try to use single daily dosing – divided dosing complicates serum level assessment and may increase the risk of renal toxicity.
- The serum lithium concentration level should be determined after 5–7 days, and the dose adjusted to achieve a value between 0.5 and 1.0 mmol/L.
- Concentrations between 0.8 and 1.0 mmol/L are usually needed for the acute treatment of mania. For prophylaxis, some patients may achieve good therapeutic results with concentrations as low as 0.4 mmol/L.

Monitoring treatment

- Mood should be monitored conscientiously (a mood diary may be helpful).
- Ask about adherence at each assessment.
- Weigh regularly.
- A reasonable schedule for blood monitoring is:
  - serum lithium level every 3 months
  - renal function every 6 months
  - thyroid function every 6 months–1 year.
- ECG if there are cardiac concerns.
- If it becomes necessary to discontinue lithium, this should be done slowly in an effort to reduce the likelihood of rebound episodes of illness.

Use in pregnancy and lactation

- Lithium has been reported to induce teratogenic defects in <11% of births, most commonly Ebstein's anomaly.
- If lithium use is necessary during pregnancy, close monitoring is advised, as is liaison with the obstetrician.
- Lithium should be stopped at the onset of labour and reintroduced in the first week postpartum.
- Lithium is excreted into breast milk, and so breastfeeding is not advised. If it is undertaken, careful monitoring of the mother's lithium concentration to keep in the lower therapeutic range is recommended.

Adverse effects of lithium

See Table 5.2. Many of the adverse effects are related to serum concentration and may be minimised if levels are kept below 0.8 mmol/L.

Table 5.2 Adverse effects of lithium

Renal (see text for discussion)
Thirst, polydipsia, polyuria
Impaired renal tubular function (5–10%)
Impaired glomerular function (possible)

Gastrointestinal symptoms
Nausea
Diarrhoea

Weight gain

Nervous system
Mild impairment of attention and memory
Tremor

Skin
Precipitates or worsens disorder (e.g. psoriasis, eczema)

Cardiac
T-wave flattening/inversion on ECG in 30% of patients

Thyroid

Hypothyroidism and nontoxic goitre (5%)
Transient hyperthyroidism (rare)

Haematological
Leucocytosis

Effects on renal function

- Lithium inhibits the action of antidiuretic hormone on the kidney and reduces the ability to concentrate urine, causing polyuria (and consequent thirst/polydipsia):
  - paradoxically this may be improved by treatment with the diuretic amiloride.
- The long-term effects of lithium on renal function are controversial:
  - polyuria does not predict lasting renal damage
  - although an early, uncontrolled, study found that 21% of patients who had been treated with lithium for more than 15 years had a reduced glomerular filtration rate, subsequent controlled studies demonstrated few differences between treated and untreated patients with respect to renal pathology.

Lithium toxicity

Lithium has a low and narrow therapeutic index – hence the need for regular monitoring. Signs of toxicity appear generally at levels above 1.3 mmol/L, although they can occur within the 'therapeutic range' in some individuals.

- Early features include:
  - exacerbation of existing side-effects
  - nausea, vomiting, diarrhoea
  - tremor.
- As toxicity develops further:
  - disorientation
  - dysarthria
  - convulsions
  - coma
  - death from cardiac effects or pulmonary complications.
- Treatment of lithium toxicity:
  - lithium toxicity represent a potentially serious and life-threatening medical emergency
  - admission may be required, for rehydration and the administration of anticonvulsants, depending on severity
  - haemodialysis may be necessary where serum levels exceed 3.0 mmol/L, coma supervenes, or there is no response to supportive measures over 24 hours.

Drug interactions with lithium

See Table 5.3.

Mortality of treated patients

- Bipolar illness carries an excess mortality.
- Lithium treatment reduces the standardised mortality rate to a level similar to the general population.
- It is estimated to increase life expectancy by about 7 years.
- The increased mortality rate returns after stopping treatment.

Table 5.3   Drug interactions with lithium

Increased lithium levels	CNS toxicity
Diuretics	Antidepressants
Nonsteroidal anti-inflammatory drugs (NSAIDs)	Antipsychotics
	Antihypertensives
Angiotensin-converting enzyme (ACE) inhibitors	General anaesthetics(?)

Other indications

- Adjunct to antidepressants in depression.
- Prevention of puerperal psychosis.
- Prophylaxis in schizoaffective disorder and cyclical schizophrenia.
- Adjunct to antipsychotics in schizophrenia.
- Reduction in impulsivity.
- Reversal of neutropenia.

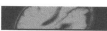 ## Anticonvulsants

Background

- The use of anticonvulsants in affective disorder is increasing. However, the mood-stabilising properties of anticonvulsants may not be mediated by the same mechanisms that mediate seizure control in epilepsy.
- The use of anticonvulsants in bipolar disorder has led to speculation about the possibility of a common pathophysiology between epilepsy and severe psychotic disorder. Processes that appear to be similar to kindling phenomena occur in the natural history of bipolar and unipolar affective disorders. Most anticonvulsant drugs with mood-stabilising properties also inhibit the electrically induced kindling of seizure activity in animals.
- The precise pharmacological properties that account for their efficacy is uncertain. In general, such drugs enhance the actions of γ-aminobutyric acid (GABA) and thus strengthen inhibitory circuits in the CNS. It is possible that their therapeutic actions are mediated through effects on membrane excitability.
- The antisuicidal effects seen with lithium do not appear to apply to anticonvulsants.
- Electroconvulsive therapy (ECT), which is also a potent anticonvulsant, has powerful antidepressive and antimanic actions.

Sodium valproate

- This is available in different formulations. Valproate semisodium (divalproex sodium in the USA) is a mixture of sodium valproate and valproic acid and is now licensed in the UK for the treatment of acute mania.
- It is the most frequently prescribed 'mood stabiliser' in the USA.
- It is increasingly used in Europe.
- It is no longer restricted to patients who have failed to respond to or are intolerant of lithium, but is increasingly being used as first-line monotherapy.

Mode of action

- Enhances GABAergic function.
- Inhibits GABA aminotransferase (transaminase) (GABA-T).
- Increases GABA binding in some brain structures, most notably the hippocampus.
- Like lithium, inhibits the formation of protein kinase C (PKC).
- Reduces the action of NA at α_2-adrenoceptors.
- May antagonise the functional effects of DA.

Indications

- Increasing use as a first-line antimanic agent.
- Treatment-refractory mania.
- Rapid-cycling bipolar disorder.
- Most effective in nonpsychotic patients.
- Although promising, further data are required before definitive statements can be made about the value of valproate in prophylaxis.
- In epilepsy, valproate is used to treat primary generalised seizures, generalised absences and myoclonic seizures.

Adverse effects

See Table 5.4.

Table 5.4 Adverse effects of valproate	
Nervous system	**Reproductive**
Tremor	Possibly polycystic ovaries and infertility in women
Liver	
Hepatotoxicity	**Teratogenic effects**
	Heart
Gastrointestinal	Neural tube
Nausea	Lip and palate
Vomiting	
	Effects on children exposed in pregnancy
Blood dyscrasias	Cognitive impairment
Weight gain	
Alopecia	

Valproate use in practice

- Monitoring of clinical condition, especially mood and weight, is important.
- There is evidence for some dose-response in the treatment of mania and loading doses can be considered to speed response in severe illness. It is unclear whether serum concentrations are a useful guide to dose, but may be helpful in cases of poor response/compliance.
- Valproate semisodium and other valproate preparations do not have the same dose equivalence (higher bioavailability with valproate semisodium).
- There is no compelling evidence for claims of significantly greater tolerability of valproate semisodium over sodium valproate.
- It is recommended that liver function be assessed before initiation, in the 6 months after, and if there are clinical concerns or if surgery is planned. Platelet and clotting function should be assessed if there are concerns and before surgery.
- Careful thought should be given to the use of valproate in women of child-bearing age (forthcoming guidance from the National Institute for Clinical Excellence (NICE) is likely to recommend that it should not routinely be given):
  - contraception should be used
  - folate supplementation should be considered
  - valproate is contraindicated in pregnancy because of adverse effect on the foetus and child.

Carbamazepine

Mode of action

- The mechanism of the therapeutic effect of carbamazepine is unknown, but it has effects on ion channels, some benzodiazepine receptors, and $GABA_B$ and adenosine receptors.
- Carbamazepine in licensed in the UK for the prophylaxis of bipolar disorder unresponsive to lithium.

Indications

- The evidence base for the efficacy of carbamazepine in treating bipolar depression and in prophylaxis is limited. Recently, a delayed-release formulation has been shown to be effective in the acute treatment of mania and mixed affective states. In maintenance studies, it appears less effective than lithium in preventing relapse.
- Limited evidence suggests that carbamazepine may be effective in treatment-resistant mania and treatment-resistant schizophrenia.
- It is used as an adjunct to lithium in the prophylaxis of bipolar affective disorder, and has been considered to have particular value in rapid-cycling bipolar disorder.

- There is no good evidence for a relationship between serum carbamazepine concentrations and efficacy. Most studies have used 600 mg daily or above.
- Although the drug enjoys a reputation for efficacy in recurrent unipolar illness and treatment-resistant depressive disorder, there is little convincing evidence to support this.
- In epilepsy, carbamazepine is used for partial or generalised tonic–clonic seizures.

Adverse effects

- Although widely regarded by British psychiatrists as a 'safer' alternative to lithium, carbamazepine has a range of potentially serious side-effects, and patient tolerance is poor (Table 5.3). Many of the autoimmune effects are thought to be related to the metabolite carbamazepine-10,11-epoxide.
- Weight gain appears less of a problem than with lithium or valproate.
- Clinical advice and monitoring for blood, hepatic and skin disorders are recommended, but the practical benefit of routine blood monitoring (i.e full blood count and liver function tests) has not been established.

Interactions

Carbamazepine has important pharmacokinetic interactions:

- It induces the metabolism of:
  - anticoagulants
  - antidepressants
  - antipsychotics
  - oral contraceptives (leading to contraceptive failure)
  - steroids.
- Other interactions occur with alcohol, analgesics, antibacterials, Ca^{2+} channel blockers and ulcer-healing drugs.

Table 5.5   Adverse effects of carbamazepine

CNS	Gastrointestinal
Headache	Nausea
Dizziness	Vomiting
Drowsiness	
Diplopia	Blood dyscrasias
	Skin rashes
Liver	
Elevation of hepatic enzymes	Teratogenic effects
Hepatitis	Possibly related to folate deficiency
Cholestatic jaundice	

Oxcarbazepine

- This has similar indications to carbamazepine in epilepsy.
- It is related to carbamazepine and has a common active metabolite, 10,11-dihydroxycarbamazepine.
- Compared with carbamazepine:
  - it is not metabolised to carbamazepine-10,11-epoxide and lacks the same propensity to cause autoimmune reactions and rashes
  - it causes less hepatic enzyme induction.
- There is a small controlled trial suggesting antimanic efficacy, but only limited open-study evidence in prophylaxis, and its place in the treatment of bipolar disorder is unclear.

Lamotrigine

- This is effective as augmentation therapy for patients with refractory epilepsy.
- It has a novel mechanism of action, stabilising neuronal membranes and reducing the release of excitatory amino acids (particularly glutamate) by blocking voltage-dependent Na^+ channels.
- It has been shown to be antidepressant in bipolar depression as monotherapy.
- It has shown efficacy in rapid-cycling bipolar disorder, and prevents relapse into bipolar depression after index episodes of both mania and bipolar depression, where it may be more effective than lithium.
- It appears to lack antimanic efficacy.
- Evidence is lacking that it is effective in treating unipolar depression.
- It can cause severe rash and Stevens–Johnson syndrome. The risk is reduced by very slow dose titration.
- Its metabolism is inhibited by sodium valproate, so even slower dose titration and lower final doses are required in patients on valproate.

Other anticonvulsants

Topiramate

- This new anticonvulsant drug is used as adjunctive therapy for partial onset seizures.
- It enhances GABA activity and blocks glutamate at non-N-methyl-D-aspartate (NMDA) receptors.
- Preliminary open observations of adjunctive topiramate treatment suggested that it may have antimanic or anticycling effects in some patients with bipolar disorder, including those who are treatment-resistant.
- However, it has not shown antimanic efficacy in controlled trials.
- Adverse effects include cognitive impairment (especially concentration and memory), anorexia, dizziness, sedation, visual and gait problems. It causes weight loss, which may be perceived as desirable by the patient.

Gabapentin

- This is in use as augmentation therapy in patients with partial seizures resistant to conventional therapies.
- It is structurally related to GABA, with an unknown mechanism of action. One possibility is through interaction with Ca^{2+} channels.
- It has been of particular interest because it possesses a wide therapeutic index and a relatively benign side-effect profile.
- Side-effects reported with gabapentin are transient and minor, the most common being somnolence, dizziness, ataxia and fatigue. It is not associated with hepatic or haematological problems.
- The use of gabapentin in rapid-cycling bipolar disorder, mania and bipolar depression has been suggested by open trials, but these findings have not been replicated in two randomised controlled trials.
- It is effective against anxiety symptoms in bipolar disorder.

Tiagabine

- This novel anticonvulsant, used as adjunctive treatment for partial seizures, reduces the reuptake of GABA into neuronal and glial cells.
- Elevated brain levels of GABA have been reported in patients with euthymic bipolar disorder using nuclear magnetic resonance spectroscopy, and therefore in theory this may be reversed by tiagabine.
- Preliminary case reports have yielded conflicting results.

Levetiracetam

- This novel anticonvulsant is used as adjunctive therapy for partial-onset seizures with unknown mechanism of action.
- There is equivocal open evidence in mania.

Zonisamide

- This novel anticonvulsant is used as adjunctive therapy for partial-onset seizures.
- It blocks Na^+ and Ca^{2+} channels and is a weak carbonic anhydrase inhibitor. It facilitiates DA and 5-HT function.
- It is currently under investigation in bipolar disorder.
- It causes weight loss when used in adjunctive therapy.

Antipsychotics (See Chapter 3)

- Typical and atypical antipsychotics are widely used in bipolar disorder.
- Antipsychotics are effective antimanic agents. Traditionally, they have been first-line agents in acute mania in Europe, whereas lithium, anticonvulsants and benzodiazepines have been preferred in the USA.

- Side-effects associated with older typical antipsychotics, and concern that they may cause depression, have meant that their use has been discouraged in prophylaxis.
- According to evidence from recent randomised controlled trials of atypical antipsychotics:
  - acute antimanic effects have been confirmed for all that have been studied (no trials with amisulpride and zotepine)
  - acute antidepressant efficacy in bipolar depression has been demonstrated for quetiapine and, to a lesser extent, olanzapine. Combining olanzapine with fluoxetine appears more effective, and this combination (Symbyax) is licensed in the USA for bipolar depression
  - olanzapine has been shown to have efficacy in prophylaxis, and it has now been licensed in the UK for the prophylaxis of bipolar disorder following its use for the acute treatment of mania. The term 'mood stabiliser' is increasingly being applied to atypical antipsychotics used in this way.

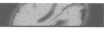 # Antidepressants (see Chapter 4)

- The use of antidepressants has generally been discouraged because of their ability to switch patients into mania – hence they are not viewed as 'mood stabilisers'.
- In practice, antidepressants are used relatively frequently because of the difficulty in treating bipolar depression. A recent meta-analysis of 12 studies supports their short-term efficacy.
- Switch rates appear highest with tricyclic antidepressants (TCAs), monoamine oxidase inhibitors (MAOIs) and dual-action reuptake inhibitors such as venlafaxine, and lowest with specific serotonin reuptake inhibitors (SSRIs), which are the preferred group if an antidepressant is indicated.
- Antidepressants should not be used in bipolar disorder without concomitant use of an antimanic agent.
- The role of antidepressants is being re-evaluated. Good evidence for benefit in prophylaxis of depressive relapse is lacking, and the routine long-term use of antidepressants is not recommended, although it may be beneficial in some individuals with bipolar disorder.

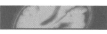 # Benzodiazepines (BDZs) (see Chapter 6)

- Although BDZs are useful in the adjunctive treatment of manic excitement and agitation, there is no evidence that they treat the underlying mood disorder.
- They are used in the USA in combination with lithium or valproate in preference to antipsychotics for the treatment of less severe acute mania.

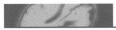 Treatment issues

- The treatment of bipolar disorder is relatively under-researched compared with schizophrenia and depression – in particular with regard to the treatment of bipolar II disorder and bipolar spectrum disorders.
- Treatment is complicated by the often chaotic nature of the illness, with different phases and presentations.
- Continuing symptoms and impaired functioning are common between major relapses.
- Only a minority of patients can be maintained on a single agent such as lithium, but at present there is limited evidence about the most effective way to combine different agents and the place of antidepressants in treatment.
- In the UK, NICE has given guidance supporting the use of olanzapine and valproate semisodium in acute mania.
- The British Association for Psychopharmacology (BAP) has published evidence-based guidelines for the treatment of bipolar disorder.
- NICE guidelines on the treatment of bipolar disorder are in their second public consultation at the time of writing.

 Guidelines

Goodwin GM, for the Consensus Group of the British Association for Psychopharmacology. Evidence-based guidelines for treating bipolar disorder: recommendations from the British Association for Psychopharmacology. J Psychopharmacol 2003; 17:149–73 (available at http://www.bap.org.uk) (Gives a good review of the treatment evidence)

National Institute for Health and Clinical Excellence. Clinical Guideline (Second Consultation). Bipolar disorder: the management of bipolar disorder in adults, children and adolescents, in primary and secondary care, 2006 http://www.nice.org.uk/page.aspx?o=guidelines.inprogress

National Institute for Clinical Excellence Technology Appraisal Guidance 66. Olanzapine and valproate semisodium in the treatment of acute mania associated with bipolar I disorder, 2003. http://www.nice.org.uk/page.aspx?o=appraisals.completed

Scottish Intercollegiate Guidelines Network National Clinical Guideline 82. Bipolar Affective Disorder, 2005. http://www.sign.ac.uk/guidelines/published/index.html

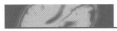 References

Key references

Achieving success in the management of bipolar disorder: Is lithium enough? A series of articles on lithium and alternatives in treating bipolar disorder in J Clin Psychiatry 2003; 64 (Suppl 5)

Bauer M, Dopfmer S. Lithium augmentation in treatment-resistant depression: meta-analysis of placebo-controlled studies. J Clin Psychopharmacol 1999; 19:427–34

Coryell W, Winokur G, Solomon D et al. Lithium and recurrence in a long-term follow-up of bipolar affective disorder. Psychol Med 1997; 27:281–9

Gijsman HJ, Geddes JR, Rendell JM, et al. Antidepressants for bipolar depression: a systematic review of randomized, controlled trials. Am J Psychiatry 2004 161:1537–47

Lenox RH, McNamara RK, Papke RL, Manji HK. Neurobiology of lithium: an update. J Clin Psychiatry 2000; 61:5–15

Manji H, Lenox R. Signaling: cellular insights into the pathophysiology of bipolar disorder. Biol Psychiatry 2000; 48:518–30

Thase M, Sachs G. Bipolar depression: pharmacotherapy and related therapeutic strategies. Biol Psychiatry 2000; 48:558–72

Tondo L, Hennen J, Baldessarini RJ. Lower suicide risk with long-term lithium treatment in major affective illness: a meta-analysis. Acta Psychiatr Scand 2001; 104:163–72

Yonkers KA, Wisner KL, Stowe Z et al Management of bipolar disorder during pregnancy and the postpartum period. Am J Psychiatry. 2004 161:608–20

Young AH, Macritchie KA, Calabrese JR. Treatment of bipolar affective disorder. New drug treatments are emerging, but more clinical evidence is required. BMJ 2000; 321:1302–3

Further reading

Drevets W, Gadde K, Krishnan K. Neuroimaging studies of mood disorders. In: (Charney D, Nestler E, Bunney B, eds). Neurobiology of Mental Illness. Oxford: Oxford University Press, 1999; 394–418

Gitlin M. Treatment-resistant bipolar disorder. Mol Psychiatry 2006; Epub ahead of print

Goodwin F, Ghaemi S. The impact of the discovery of lithium on psychiatric thought and practice in the USA and Europe. Aust NZ J Psychiatry 1999; 33:S54–64

Hasler G, Drevets WC, Gould TD et al, Toward constructing an endophenotype strategy for bipolar disorders. Biol Psychiatry 2006; 11(3):227–40

Post R. Mood disorders: treatment of bipolar disorders. In: (Sadock B, Sadock V, eds). Kaplan & Sadock's Comprehensive Textbook of Psychiatry. New York: Williams & Wilkins, 2000; 1385–430

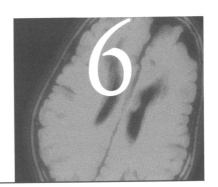

Anxiolytics

Stephen J Cooper

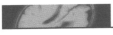 History

- *Pre-benzodiazepine era*: Bromides, chloral and paraldehyde were introduced in the 19th century and barbiturates, and meprobamate in the 20th century, but there were problems with the low therapeutic index. Barbiturates predominated until the introduction of benzodiazepines (BDZs).
- *Benzodiazepine era*: Chlordiazepoxide (1960) was followed by diazepam, with a rapid growth in use, peaking about 1979. These had a higher therapeutic index than barbiturates, but addiction and withdrawal problems at the usual therapeutic doses were fully recognised in 1981, leading to reduced prescribing (Table 6.1):
  - in 1978, 10% of men and 20% of women were given a BDZ: 15% for >4 weeks, 1.5% for >1 year. For anxiety, peak prescribing was in the age range 50–65 years; for hypnotics, the peak prescribing was for patients aged 65 years or older. Long-term use was associated with the elderly, and with multiple, chronic physical disorders
  - hypnotic prescriptions have remained fairly constant at 10–12 million per annum.
- *Post-benzodiazepine era*: Alternatives to benzodiazepines were developed that are less/nonaddictive (e.g. serotonergic drugs, BDZ partial agonists, γ-aminobutyric acid (GABA)/peptidergic drugs), but BDZs remain frequently used.

Table 6.1 Benzodiazepine prescribing in the UK

Year	UK prescriptions for hypnotics and tranquillisers	Comments
1960	27 million	15 million barbiturates
1974	40 million	25 million benzodiazepines
1979	31 million	Few for barbiturates
1990	16 million	12 million hypnotics

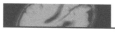 ## Neurobiology

Brain aversion system

- Periaqueductal grey (PAG):
    - brainstem area
    - linked to stereotyped, 'hard-wired' responses of fight or flight
    - panic attacks likely to be linked to activation of PAG: spontaneous panics may originate at this level.
- Medial hypothalamus:
    - autonomic and endocrine components of anxiety response.
- Amygdala:
    - important role in classical conditioning and coordinating/integrating fear responses
    - response to cues and close threat (e.g. startle reactions), with inputs from thalamus
    - likely to be involved in phobias and post-traumatic stress disorder (PTSD).
- Septohippocampal system:
    - role in context of anxiety and inhibition of behaviour
    - likely role in avoidance and anticipatory anxiety.
- Temporal and prefrontal cortex:
    - higher-order processing, including of social situations
    - likely role in anticipatory and socially induced anxiety.

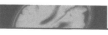 ## Neurochemical theories

Noradrenaline (NA)

- Stimulation of the major brain NA nucleus, the locus ceruleus (LC) in animals gives an anxiety-like state.
- Physiological symptoms of anxiety in humans are consistent with adrenergic overactivity.
- Yohimbine (α_2-antagonist) infusion increases NA release and causes panic in panic disorder patients, but has little effect in non-anxious subjects.
- Clonidine (α_2-agonist) infusion causes decreased NA release and may decrease anxiety in some situations.
- β-adrenoceptor antagonists reduce physiological symptoms of anxiety.

Serotonin (5-HT)

- 5-HT_{1A} partial agonists (e.g. buspirone) can decrease anxiety in generalised anxiety disorder (GAD) but are not effective in panic disorder.

- Some 5-HT$_2$ agonists (e.g. *m*-chlorophenylpiperazine) are anxiogenic.
- Selective serotonin reuptake inhibitors (SSRIs) are effective in treating a wide range of anxiety disorders – GAD, panic disorder, social anxiety disorder, PTSD, obsessive–compulsive disorder (OCD) – but can make anxiety symptoms worse in the initial phase of treatment of panic disorder.
- 5-HT has a complex role in anxiety:
  - in animal models of anxiety, the effect of 5-HT depends on the model and anxiety situation being examined
  - 5-HT acts at different levels of the brain aversion system, inhibiting the brainstem hard-wired panic system but increasing anxiety in temporal lobe structures involved in conditioned/generalised anxiety
  - human studies suggest that 5-HT stimulation reduces panic anxiety but increases generalised anxiety.
- In addition, there is 'crosstalk' between neurotransmitters, e.g. according to one theory: ↑5-HT release → ↑frontal cortex stimulation → ↓activity of GABA projection to LC → ↑LC firing.

GABA

- BDZs (which enhance GABA function) are effective in treatment of anxiety.
- Pentylenetetrazol (an inhibitor of the GABA$_A$–BDZ receptor) causes extreme anxiety symptoms and seizures.
- Flumazenil (a BDZ inhibitor) may cause panic in panic patients, but not in non-anxious subjects (which possibly indicates an abnormality of BDZ receptor sensitivity in panic disorder).
- BDZ receptor numbers (measured by positron emission tomography (PET) studies of flumazenil binding) are reduced by 20% in panic disorder patients.
- Mice genetically altered to have only 50% of the γ_2 subunits (linked to the BDZ-binding site) in GABA$_A$–BDZ receptors (receptor 'knockout') have the behavioural equivalent of anxiety.
- The effect of BDZs may involve acting on receptors on monoamine neurons, e.g. brainstem and LC, leading to reduced NA and 5-HT neuronal firing.

Carbon dioxide (CO$_2$)

- Increased sensitivity to inhaled CO$_2$ in panic disorder leads to panic anxiety (but, paradoxically, voluntary hyperventilation, causing hypocapnia, can also induce panic).
- Lactate infusion (possibly by altering acid–base balance) provokes panic in anxious patients but not in controls.
- This finding is consistent with possible alteration of brainstem sensitivity to CO$_2$.

Cholecystokinin (CCK)

- Infusion of CCK4 and pentagastrin (agonists at CCK_B receptors) induces panic in humans.
- CCK_B receptor antagonists are anxiolytic in some animal models.

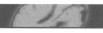 # Drug treatment of anxiety

- The anxiety disorders comprise a group of disorders with anxiety as a cardinal feature. There is considerable overlap with depression, and 'mixed anxiety and depression' is commonly found in primary care.
- In the UK, the National Institute for Clinical Excellence (NICE) guidelines for treating panic disorder and GAD were published in 2004, and those for PTSD and OCD in 2005:
    - these guidelines emphasise psychological treatment in the first line
    - they are constrained by gaps in the evidence, and are not entirely pharmacologically consistent.
- Table 6.2 summarises the placebo-controlled randomised controlled trial (RCT) evidence for drug efficacy in the anxiety disorders.
- Drug treatment:
    - often brings about improvement rather than cure in anxiety disorders
    - usually needs to be combined with psychological/behavioural management strategies, even if not formal psychotherapy
    - treatment trials need to be of adequate duration to assess benefit (typically at least 12 weeks)
    - relapse/worsening is likely on discontinuation, and therefore treatment needs to be continued for at least 6–12 months after improvement, often longer.
- There is no good evidence that specific phobias respond to drug treatment.

Benzodiazepines

- BDZs act at the $GABA_A$–BDZ receptor complex (see Chapter 1 and Fig. 6.1).
- Endogenous ligands have been identified, but their functional status is unknown.
- The $GABA_A$–BDZ complex consists of five subunits from seven families of subunits (α, β, γ, δ, ε, π, ρ), each of which contains a number of subtypes of units. The most common type of $GABA_A$–BDZ receptor (50% of the total) contains two α_1, two β_2 and one γ_2 subunit (see Fig. 6.1 and Fig. 1.11), arranged around the Cl^- ion channel.
- GABA is the main inhibitory transmitter in the central nervous system (CNS). Two GABA molecules are required to increase Cl^- ion channel conductance (by increasing the time for which the channel is open). This reduces the likelihood of an action potential.

Table 6.2 Summary of treatments with placebo-controlled trial efficacy for the pharmacological treatment of anxiety disorders. (Based on BAP guidelines for the pharmacological treatment of anxiety disorders: Baldwin et al 2005)

	GAD	Panic disorder	Social phobia	OCD	PTSD
Acute efficacy	SSRI[a], imipramine, venlafaxine, BDZ[a], buspirone, hydroxyzine, pregabalin, trifluoperazine	SSRI[a], imipramine, clomipramine, venlafaxine, reboxetine, BDZ[a], sodium valproate	SSRI[a], venlafaxine, phenelzine, moclobemide, gabapentin, pregabalin, olanzapine	SSRI[a], imipramine, clomipramine	SSRI[a], imipramine, amitriptyline, venlafaxine, mirtazapine, phenelzine, brofaromine, BDZ[a], lamotrigine
Longer-term efficacy	SSRI[a], venlafaxine	SSRI[a], imipramine, clomipramine, BDZ[a]	SSRI[a], venlafaxine, phenelzine, moclobemide	SSRI[a], clomipramine	SSRI[a]
Efficacy after non-response	—	SSRI[a,b]	—	BDZ[a], haloperidol[c], risperidone[c], quetiapine[c], pindolol[c]	olanzapine[c], risperidone[c]

GAD, generalised anxiety disorder; OCD, obsessive–compulsive disorder; PTSD, post-traumatic stress disorder; SSRI, selective serotonin reuptake inhibitor; BDZ, benzodiazepine.

[a] Evidence for individual drugs within the class varies between disorders.
[b] After non-response to cognitive–behavioural therapy.
[c] Augmentation of ongoing treatment.

- The BDZ binding site is at the junction between the α_1 and γ_2 subunits (see Fig. 6.1).
- When a BDZ occupies its own receptor, it enhances the action of GABA at its receptor, resulting in greater flow of Cl^- into the neuron.
- If GABA is absent or the receptor is blocked (e.g. by bicuculline) then BDZs on their own will have no effect, making them relatively safe in overdose (cf. barbiturates, which can open the channel in the absence of GABA, resulting in respiratory depression).
- Type I BDZ receptors are mainly found in the cerebellum, and are related to induction and maintenance of sleep, whereas type II BDZ receptors tend to be found in the spinal cord and limbic regions, and are associated with muscle relaxant, anxiolytic and anticonvulsant effects.
- Newer hypnotic drugs modulate the $GABA_A$–BDZ receptor complex, but have pharmacodynamic differences to BDZ:

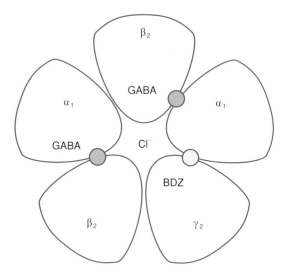

Figure 6.1   GABA$_A$–benzodiazepine (BDZ) receptor complex, showing subunits and binding sites of ligands (binding sites for γ-aminobutyric acid (GABA) and BDZ are shown by filled circles).

- – zolpidem (an imadazopyridine) and zaleplon (a pyrazolopyrimidine) are relatively selective for the type I receptor
- – zopiclone (a cyclopyrrolone) binds to a different site on the GABA$_A$–BDZ receptor complex from standard BDZs and zolpidem.

Agonist/inverse agonist effects (Table 6.3)

- ▪ BDZ effects are through modulation of GABA function. BDZs are unusual in having inhibitory and stimulatory effects on GABA function.
- ▪ Full agonists (e.g. diazepam) and partial agonists at the BDZ receptor act to *enhance* the action of GABA.
- ▪ Full and partial inverse agonists *inhibit* the action of GABA. They act in the opposite way to a typical BDZ and reduce Cl⁻ influx. There are no clinically useful drugs in this category at present. However, in patients with panic disorder, flumazenil may act like a partial inverse agonist and cause an increase in anxiety symptoms.
- ▪ Neutral antagonists occupy the BDZ receptor and prevent agonists or inverse agonists interacting with it. Flumazenil does this under most circumstances.

Effects of benzodiazepines (Table 6.4)

- ▪ There is little direct effect on autonomic, cardiovascular or respiratory function unless given intravenously.
- ▪ There is no hepatic enzyme induction.

Table 6.3 Range of effects possible for drugs active at the BDZ receptor

Full agonist	Partial agonist	Neutral antagonist	Partial inverse agonist	Full inverse agonist
Action				
Sedative	Mild sedation			
Anxiolytic	Mild anxiolytic	No effect of	Anxiogenic	Anxiogenic
Anticonvulsant	Anticonvulsant	its own		Proconvulsant
Example				
Diazepam	Clonazepam	Flumazenil	FG7142 (Flumazenil in patients with panic disorder)	Ethyl-β-carboline-3-carboxylate (β-CCE)

Table 6.4 Principal actions of benzodiazepines

Action	Use
Anxiolytic	Anxiety disorders, alcohol withdrawal, premedication in anaesthesia
Hypnotic	
Anticonvulsant	Sleep disorder
Muscle relaxant	Epilepsy, myoclonus, alcohol withdrawal
Amnesic	Muscle spasticity, akathisia
Impairment of psychomotor function	Premedication

Clinical efficacy of benzodiazepines in psychiatric disorders

- Sleep:
  - pharmacokinetic properties are important (see below); shorter elimination half-life compounds preferred
  - newer compounds with different pharmacodynamics to classical BDZs (zolpidem, zopiclone, zaleplon) are claimed to cause less dependence/withdrawal
  - very short-half-life compounds (zaleplon) are only useful for sleep induction and not sleep maintenance
  - in the UK, NICE (2004) has given guidance that there is no compelling evidence to distinguish between the newer compounds and shorter-acting BDZ hypnotics. This is disputed by some user groups and experts due to the longer half-lives of BDZ hypnotics (see Table 6.7).

- Anxiety disorders:
  - longer-half-life drugs are indicated; short-half-life drugs are more prone to withdrawal problems
  - BDZs are effective in 'core' anxiety disorders; efficacy seems to be maintained for many patients with GAD and panic disorder; some may develop tolerance
  - BDZs are not believed to be effective as primary treatment for longer-term treatment of other anxiety disorders such as social phobia, specific phobias, OCD and PTSD, but there have been few long-term clinical trials (see Table 6.2).
- Alcohol withdrawal and epilepsy:
  - longer-half-life drugs are indicated.

Adverse effects of benzodiazepines (Table 6.5)

- The context of use determines whether some of these (e.g. sedation, amnesia) are wanted or unwanted.

Pharmacokinetics (Tables 6.6 and 6.7)

- Many BDZs undergo phase I metabolism to produce active metabolites that:
  - generally have a much longer elimination half-life than the parent compound
  - lead to prolonged effects as their plasma concentration gradually rises
  - are often largely responsible for 'hangover' effects when a BDZ is used regularly as a hypnotic
  - may contribute to confusion in susceptible subjects (e.g. the elderly).
- Compounds lacking phase I metabolism with short elimination half-lives are preferred as hypnotics (but note nitrazepam in Table 6.7, which has historically been used as a hypnotic).

Table 6.5 Main adverse effects of benzodiazepines

Frequency	Adverse effect
Common	Drowsiness, dizziness, psychomotor impairment
Occasional	Dry mouth, blurred vision, gastrointestinal upset, headache; increased risk of falls in the elderly
Rare	Amnesia, restlessness, disinhibition, skin rash, eosinophilia, respiratory arrest (parenteral administration)

Table 6.6 Main pharmacokinetic properties of benzodiazepines, using diazepam as an example

Bioavailability	Almost complete with oral dose
Peak concentration	30–90 minutes after single dose
Protein binding	95%
Renal excretion	Negligible for unchanged drug
Metabolism	Phase I to active metabolite Phase II for inactivation
Elimination half-life	Young adults: 20 hours Elderly: 30–100 hours Phase I metabolite, desmethyldiazepam: 30–90 hours

Table 6.7 Pharmacokinetic parameters for a number of BDZs and similar compounds

Drug	Absorption	Half-life (parent drug) (h)	Metabolic phases	Half-life (active metabolite) (h)	Clinical use
Diazepam	Rapid	20–100	I+II	30–90	Anxiolytic
Alprazolam	Intermediate	5–15	I+II	Very low concentration	Antipanic
Lorazepam	Intermediate	10–20	II only	None	Anxiolytic
Nitrazepam	Intermediate	24	I+II	30–90	Hypnotic
Flurazepam	Rapid	2	I+II	30–100	Hypnotic
Temazepam	Slow	10	II only	None	Hypnotic
Zolpidem	Rapid	2	II only	None	Hypnotic
Zopiclone	Rapid	4	I+II	3–6	Hypnotic
Zaleplon	Rapid	1	II only	None	Hypnotic

Tolerance (see also Chapter 2)

▪ Increased rapid eye movement sleep amount and intensity (REM rebound) is one example of the development of tolerance to the effects of BDZs when used as hypnotics:
  - BDZs reduce REM sleep from 25% to 10–15% of total sleep time at night, with tolerance occurring within about 2 weeks (REM% returns to normal)
  - sudden discontinuation of BDZ leads to a rebound increase in REM sleep, resulting in periods of waking through the night (can take up to 6 weeks to return to normal)
  - this leads to the patient believing that they must continue the hypnotic drug and to the development of physical dependence.

- Tolerance to different effects of BDZs is not entirely clear – evidence suggests the following:
  - *animals*: tolerance occurs to sedation, ataxia, muscle relaxation and anticonvulsant effects, but is less clear for 'anxiolytic' effects
  - *humans*: tolerance occurs to sedation, anticonvulsant and EEG effects, but is less clear for psychomotor, anxiolytic and hypnotic effects.
- Cross-tolerance may occur to other BDZs and alcohol.
- The mechanism of tolerance with BDZs is not entirely clear, but is likely to be a combination of pharmacodynamic and cognitive/behavioural factors.

Benzodiazepine withdrawal syndrome (Table 6.8)

- This was first described fully by Petursson and Lader (1981).
- It had previously been recognised following prolonged, high-dose treatment, but they described it following shorter periods of standard doses.
- It probably affects 45% of people on cessation or dose reduction.
- Personality variables have some predictive value: it is more common in a dependent personality.

Management of benzodiazepine withdrawal syndrome

- Gradually decrease BDZ dose over 4–16 weeks.
- Transfer to longer-half-life drug, e.g. diazepam.
- β-blockers can reduce the severity of symptoms, but do not appear to improve outcome.
- Monitor for increased alcohol consumption.
- Outcome:
  - most succeed initially
  - one-third have some relapse but later succeed
  - one-third fully relapse and remain on BDZs.

Table 6.8 Symptoms of benzodiazepine withdrawal

Anxiety-type symptoms	Disturbance of perception	Severe but rare symptoms
Anxiety	Hypersensitivity to stimuli	Paranoid psychosis
Dysphoria	Abnormal bodily sensation	Depressive episode
Tremor	Sense of body sway	Seizures
Muscle pains	Depersonalisation	
Sleep disturbance	Visual disturbances	
Headache		
Nausea, anorexia		
Sweating		
Fatigue		

Toxicity in overdose

- Patients have survived overdoses of greater than 2 g. Psychomotor impairment has been detected for some weeks afterwards.
- Treatment:
    - supportive therapy and gastric lavage if appropriate
    - dialysis is probably of limited value, given the large volume of distribution of these drugs
    - flumazenil will counteract sedation, but beware of its short half-life.

Benzodiazepines in pregnancy

- There have been reports of cleft lip and cleft palate in uncontrolled studies.
- Respiratory depression has occurred in the newborns of mothers on BDZs. Developmental dysmorphism (e.g. fetal alcohol syndrome) was reported in 1987. However, this study was complicated by the mothers' alcohol use. The findings were not replicated in a 1992 study.

Place in clinical practice and prescribing guidelines

- BDZs are most effective for acute anxiety states and GAD.
- Where possible, identify causes of anxiety or insomnia, and treat these appropriately.
- Reserve BDZs for more severe symptoms.
- Use the lowest effective dose.
- Ideally, only prescribe for 2 weeks, and at most 4 weeks. Caution is needed if BDZs are considered for chronic anxiety, where prescription may be required for more than 2–4 weeks (note that this is not recommended in the NICE guidelines).
- Avoid 'repeat' prescriptions as far as possible.
- Warn patients about the possibility of dependence.

5-HT_{1A} receptor agonists

Background

- Buspirone is available (a 5-HT_{1A} receptor partial agonist). Others such as gepirone and ipsapirone have not come to market.
- Buspirone causes a complex cascade of events in the 5-HT system: initially, an effect at the somatodendritic receptor causes a decrease in 5-HT release, but the effect is mitigated by postsynaptic receptor agonism; chronic treatment (>2 weeks) results in a return to normal of 5-HT neuronal firing and release. Combined with a direct postsynaptic effect, this may lead to an overall increase in 5-HT neurotransmission.

- The elimination half-life is short (3 hours), so multiple daily dosing is necessary. The slow-release form has an effective half-life of 9 hours. The active metabolite 1-pyramidinylpiperazine (1-PP, an α_2-antagonist) may contribute to the effect of buspirone.

Efficacy

- Trials demonstrate effectiveness for GAD but not panic disorder.
- No consistent evidence for other anxiety disorders.
- Some evidence for better effect if patients have not recently been exposed to BDZs.
- Also evidence for effectiveness for depression.
- Trials of augmentation of SSRIs in depressive and anxiety disorders have not shown efficacy.

Adverse effects

- Nausea, dizziness, headache.
- No evidence of a withdrawal syndrome.
- No interaction with alcohol.

Place in clinical practice

- Used for GAD especially if associated with symptoms of depression.
- Does not appear to be as effective as BDZs and takes longer to act. Thus of little use for acute anxiety.

Antidepressants

Background

- Tricyclic antidepressants (TCAs) were used for many years in the management of anxiety, although there were no large-sized RCTs until the 1980s.
- Monoamine oxidase inhibitors (MAOIs) have been used for so-called 'atypical depression', which has had different definitions but historically includes mild/moderate depressive states with a large anxiety component (however, the DSM-IV definition does not specify anxiety; see Chapter 4).
- The efficacy of imipramine in panic disorder was used to argue for it being a distinct disorder (in the mistaken belief that panic disorder did not respond to BDZs).
- Clomipramine was the first drug demonstrated to be of benefit for OCD.
- More recently, there have been extensive trials with the SSRIs in the anxiety disorders (Table 6.2).

Mode of action and adverse effects

▦ See Chapter 4 for details of the pharmacodynamic effects of antidepressants and their adverse effects.

▦ The efficacy of antidepressants in anxiety disorders is probably related to their effects on the 5-HT system.

Efficacy (Table 6.2)

▦ RCTs have demonstrated efficacy of TCAs for anxiety associated with depression, GAD, panic disorder, OCD and PTSD. Only the more serotonergic TCAs (especially clomipramine) are effective in OCD, and possibly panic disorder.

▦ Clinical trials with SSRIs show efficacy across the range of anxiety disorders.

▦ Venlafaxine, a joint 5-HT and NA reuptake inhibitor (SNRI), has been extensively tested in GAD, with evidence of efficacy in some other anxiety disorders, as would be expected from its pharmacology:

  – for GAD, there is a possible dose-response up to 150 mg (note that NICE only recommends 75 mg)

  – in the UK, the Committee on Safety of Medicines has recommended prescribing restrictions because of cardiac concerns, although this is under appeal at the time of writing (see also Chapter 4).

▦ Other antidepressants, such as MAOIs, mirtazapine and reboxetine, have shown efficacy in some anxiety disorders (Table 6.2).

Place in clinical practice

▦ SSRIs are first-line for GAD, panic disorder, social phobia, OCD and PTSD.

▦ Serotonergic TCAs are second-line for panic disorder (clomipramine, imipramine) and OCD (clomipramine); venlafaxine is second-line for GAD.

▦ In the first 2 weeks of treatment with an SSRI, panic symptoms can worsen and may be treated with a short-term BDZ.

β-Adrenoceptor antagonists

Background

▦ A series of classical trials in the 1960s demonstrated that there was an effect on anxiety symptoms that was due to a peripheral effect (practolol) on β-adrenoceptors (use of D- and L-isomers).

▦ Anxiety associated with thyrotoxicosis was shown to respond.

▦ It is not clear if the effect is mainly through $β_1$- or $β_2$-adrenoceptors.

Efficacy

▦ Ten small studies, some placebo-controlled, consistently show benefit for situational/performance anxiety.

- Studies to date suggest only limited efficacy in GAD.
- They are ineffective in panic disorder, from limited evidence.
- They attenuate the severity of BDZ withdrawal symptoms.

Adverse effects

- May lead to hypotension from bradycardia.
- Excessive dreaming.
- Can aggravate bronchospasm, cardiac failure.
- Some observational evidence of depression of mood, but this is not consistent.

Place in clinical practice

- First-line for situational/performance anxiety.
- May help some GAD/panic disorder patients with many physiological symptoms of anxiety.
- Also of value for akathisia and lithium-induced fine tremor (not toxicity).

Antipsychotics

- These have been used from the 1950s – mainly the low-potency drugs thioridazine (but the licence is now limited to schizophrenia and requires ECG monitoring) and chlorpromazine.
    - they have tended to be used in low dose
    - their antihistaminergic actions may contribute.
- There have been very few clinical trials, and most of which were small and not placebo-controlled.
- There is, however, limited RCT evidence (Table 6.2) for:
    - olanzapine and risperidone augmentation of SSRIs in PTSD
    - haloperidol, risperidone and quetiapine augmentation of SSRIs in OCD
    - trifluoperazine in GAD
    - olanzapine in social phobia.
- With typical antipsychotics, there is a risk of extrapyramidal side-effects and, with long-term use, tardive dyskinesia.
- They are useful for short-term use in the treatment of anxiety/agitation in association with severe depressive disorder.
- In general, the place of atypical antipsychotics is not established in anxiety disorders.
- Antipsychotics should only be considered for careful augmentation treatment trials in refractory GAD, OCD and PTSD.

Other/new approaches

- The antihistamine hydroxyzine has been shown to have short-term efficacy in GAD.
- 5-HT$_2$ antagonists appear to have efficacy in GAD but not panic disorder (which they may exacerbate). No 5-HT$_2$ antagonists are marketed for anxiety disorders, but antidepressants with 5-HT$_2$ antagonism include trazodone, mirtazapine and nefazodone (now withdrawn in the UK).
- Some anticonvulsants appear to have efficacy in some anxiety disorders (Table 6.2). At least for some, this may be related to their effects on GABA.
- CCK antagonists have not shown evidence for efficacy in clinical trials. Bioavailability is a problem with these compounds.
- Corticotropin-releasing factor (CRF) can be anxiogenic, and CRF$_1$ receptor antagonists may be anxiolytic. Bioavailability is a problem with these compounds.
- Neurokinin (NK, substance P) can be anxiogenic in laboratory animals. NK$_1$ and NK$_2$ receptor antagonists are anxiolytic in some animal models, where they are not as potent as BDZs but better than SSRIs. Evidence from clinical trials in patients remains mixed.
- Pregabalin, which acts on a subunit of the voltage-gated Ca^{2+} channel, shows evidence of effect in recent clinical trials in GAD and social phobia, and has been approved for the treatment of GAD by the European Commission.
- Kava kava comes from the root of a plant in some Pacific islands. It has been used there for many generations, and has been in phase II and III clinical trials. It was available until recently as a complementary treatment, but has been withdrawn due to concerns about hepatotoxicity.

 ## Guidelines

Baldwin DS, Anderson IM, Nutt DJ et al. Evidence-based guidelines for the pharmacological treatment of anxiety disorders: recommendations from the British Association for Psychopharmacology. J. Psychopharmacol 2005 19:567–96 (Gives a good review of the evidence-base for treatment of anxiety disorders)

National Institute for Clinical Excellence. Clinical Guideline 22. Anxiety: Management of anxiety (panic disorder, with or without agoraphobia, and generalised anxiety disorder) in adults in primary, secondary and community care, 2004, http://www.nice.org.uk/page.aspx?o=guidelines.completed

National Institute for Clinical Excellence. Clinical Guideline 26. Post-traumatic stress disorder (PTSD): the management of PTSD in adults and children in primary and secondary care, 2005. http://www.nice.org.uk/page.aspx?o=guidelines.completed

National Institute for Health and Clinical Excellence. Clinical Guideline 31. Obsessive–compulsive disorder: core interventions in the treatment of obsessive–compulsive disorder

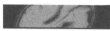

and body dysmorphic disorder, 2005. http://www.nice.org.uk/page.aspx?o=guidelines. completed

National Institute for Clinical Excellence Technology Appraisal Guidance 77. Guidance on the use of zaleplon, zolpidem and zopiclone for the short-term management of insomnia, 2004. http://www.nice.org.uk/page.aspx?o=appraisals. completed

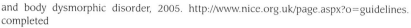

References

Key references

Granville-Grossman KL, Turner P. The effect of propranolol on anxiety. Lancet 1966; i:788–790

Klein DF. Delineation of two drug-responsive anxiety syndromes. Psychopharmacologia 1964; 5:397–408

Petursson H, Lader MH. Withdrawal from long-term benzodiazepine treatment. BMJ 1981;283:643–5

Squires RF, Braestrup C. Benzodiazepine receptors in rat brain. Nature 1977; 274:732–4

Further reading

Cooper SJ. Anxiolytics, sedatives and hypnotics. In: (King DJ, ed). Seminars in Clinical Psychopharmacology, 2nd edn. London: Gaskell, 2004

Griebel G. Is there a future for neuropeptide receptor ligands in the treatment of anxiety disorders? Pharmacol Therapeut 1999; 82:1–61 (Gives a comprehensive review of this field, but is for the seriously enthusiastic only)

Mitte K, Noack P, Steil R, Hautzinger M. A meta-analytic review of the efficacy of drug treatment in generalized anxiety disorder. J Clin Psychopharmacol 2005 25: 141–50

Paul SM. GABA and glycine. In: (Bloom FE , Kupfer DJ, eds). Psychopharmacology, the Fourth Generation of Progress New York: Raven Press, 1994: 87–94

Royal College of Psychiatrists. Benzodiazepines: risks, benefits or dependence. A re-evaluation. Council Report CR59. London: Royal College of Psychiatrists, 1997

Shiloh R, Stryjer R, Nutt D, Weizman A. Atlas of Psychiatric Pharmacotherapy, 2nd edn. London: Taylor & Francis, 2006

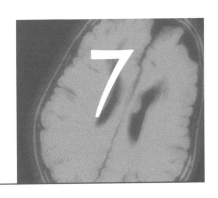

Drugs of abuse

Anne Lingford-Hughes and Mark Daglish

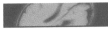

Why take drugs?

- For pleasure, to get a 'rush', euphoria, i.e. for positive reinforcement or reward.
- As anxiolytics or to overcome withdrawal, i.e. negative reinforcement.
- Because their use cannot be controlled, overwhelming urge, compulsion.

The faster the onset of the drug effects, the better the 'rush':

Slow						*Fast*
Chewing tobacco			$\rightarrow$	snuff	$\rightarrow$	cigarettes
Coca leaves	$\rightarrow$	coca paste	$\rightarrow$	cocaine	$\rightarrow$	crack cocaine
Methadone	$\rightarrow$	morphine	$\rightarrow$	snorted heroin	$\rightarrow$	intravenous heroin

History

- The pattern of drug use changes with time, depending on what is available and how much it costs.
- Many drugs that are now considered 'addictive' were introduced for medical purposes.
- Alcohol:
  - there is evidence of fermentation processes occurring approximately 7000 years ago
  - currently, it is the mostly widely used legal drug and its relative cost is decreasing.
- Opioids:
  - opium has been used medically since ancient times
  - morphine was isolated in 1805
  - methadone was first synthesised in Germany during World War II.
- Stimulants:
  - amfetamine was synthesised in the late 1880s for therapeutic purposes
  - cocaine alkaloid was first isolated in 1860 and used as a local anaesthetic

- – metamfetamine (a derivative of amfetamine) is increasingly used in the USA, UK and in other countries.
- Cannabis:
    - – its effects have been documented for many centuries
    - – its nonmedical use, for its hedonic properties, began in the early 19th century in Europe.
- Hallucinogens include both natural (psilocybin) and synthetic (lysergic acid diethylamide, LSD) compounds:
    - – the hallucinogenic powers of LSD were discovered when it was accidentally absorbed in 1943. The term 'psychedelic' was coined in the 1950s
    - – the use of psychedelic drugs predominated in the 1960s.
- Tobacco is a plant native of the American continent:
    - – it is believed to have been first used in the 1st century AD
    - – it has been smoked in Europe from around the end of the 15th century.

In conceptualizing the recreational use/misuse of drugs, different models have been applied:

- medical (disease model)
- psychological (learning theory)
- philosophical/moral.

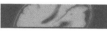

Legal issues (UK)

- The Misuse of Drugs Act 1971 relates to the manufacture, supply and possession of 'Controlled Drugs'. Drugs are ascribed to one of three classes based on the perceived harmfulness when they are misused; the penalties are set accordingly (see the British National Formulary (BNF) for the complete listing:
    - – *Class A* includes cocaine, diamorphine (heroin), dipipanone, lysergide (LSD), methadone, methylenedioxymethamfetamine (MDMA, Ecstasy, 'E'), morphine, opium, pethidine, phencyclidine and class B substances when prepared for injection.
    - – *Class B* includes oral amfetamines, barbiturates, codeine and pentazocine.
    - – *Class C* includes certain drugs related to the amfetamines (e.g. benzfetamine and chlorphentermine), buprenorphine, diethylpropion, mazindol, meprobamate, pemoline, pipradrol, most benzodiazepines (BDZs), androgenic and anabolic steroids, clenbuterol, cannabis and cannabis resin (controversially reclassified from Class B to C in 2004), and ketamine (from 2006).
- See the BNF for regulations related to prescribing of controlled drugs.

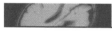

Scientific background

Drugs of abuse and dopamine (DA)

- Drugs of abuse increase DA concentration in the nucleus accumbens (NAcc) of the mesolimbic system (Figs 7.1 and 1.3):
    - – The NAcc has high levels of D_3 receptors.

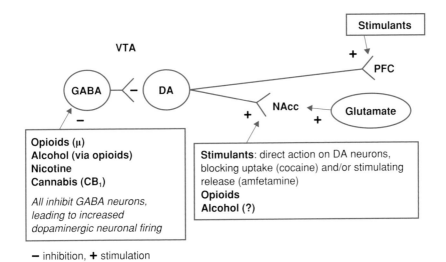

Figure 7.1 The dopamine (DA) reinforcement pathway. DA neurons in the ventral tegmental area (VTA) project to mesolimbic areas (including the nucleus accumbens, NAcc) and prefrontal cortex (PFC). GABA neurons in the VTA inhibit DA neuronal firing and can be inhibited by drugs such as opioids through μ-receptors and canabinoids through CB_1 receptors. This results in disinhibition (activation) of the DA neurons and increased release of DA in NAcc (and PFC). Stimulant drugs act directly on DA neurons in the NAcc and PFC.

- Increase in DA function is key in mediating positive reinforcement:
  - DA is increased by cocaine, amfetamine, alcohol, opiates, nicotine and cannabinoids (Fig 7.1)
  - BDZs are the only drugs of abuse not shown to significantly increase DA.
- DA release in the mesolimbic system, including the NAcc, prefrontal cortex, dorsal striatum and amygdala, is also involved in reward-related learning.
- Reduced DA concentrations are seen in withdrawal states, and are likely to be associated with depression, irritability, dysphoria.
- Sensitisation (a progressive increase in an effect of a drug with repeated administration; see Chapter 2) is associated with stimulant abuse.
- DA is modulated by opioids (Fig. 7.1). This is the pharmacological basis for the efficacy of naltrexone in the treatment of alcohol dependence.
- Glutamatergic projections from the prefrontal cortex, hippocampus, amygdala and NAcc, and in particular N-methyl-D-aspartate (NMDA) receptors, play an important role in sensitisation and reward-based learning.

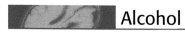 # Alcohol

Neuropharmacology

There is no 'alcohol receptor' as such. Alcohol primarily modulates ion channel function – γ-aminobutyric acid (GABA)–BDZ, NMDA, and 5-HT$_3$ receptors – and the following neurotransmitter systems are involved in mediating its effects.

Alcohol and GABA function

▦ Alcohol mediates many of its actions through modulating GABA function – it is an agonist at GABA$_A$ or GABA–BDZ receptors (see Chapters 1 and 6 for details of the GABA$_A$ receptor).

▦ Different subunits of the receptor confer different alcohol sensitivity. Recently, α_5-containing receptors have been shown to be involved with alcohol reinforcement.

▦ This varied sensitivity is a possible mechanism of vulnerability to alcoholism.

▦ Chronic alcohol exposure is associated with reduced GABA function and reduced levels of specific receptor subunits, leading to tolerance.

▦ This interaction underlies the cross-tolerance between alcohol and BDZs.

Alcohol and glutamate function

▦ Alcohol is an NMDA antagonist, causing decreased Ca^{2+} influx into neurons and decreased excitability (see Chapter 1) – this may account for its effects on memory, e.g. amnesia (blackouts).

▦ Chronic alcohol exposure increases NMDA receptor function, which leads in withdrawal to a hyperexcitable state, which is probably the mechanism underlying seizures and brain damage through excitatory neurotoxicity.

Alcohol and monoamine function

Dopamine (DA)

▦ Reduced DA responses are seen in patients with alcoholism.

▦ These reduced responses may predict relapse and be associated with depressive symptomatology – dysphoria, irritability, restlessness.

▦ An association with D_2 receptor polymorphism has been reported in some groups of alcoholics.

▦ D_2 receptor-deficient mice show a marked aversion to alcohol.

Noradrenaline (NA)

Increased activity may occur in alcohol withdrawal; however, lofexidine (an α_2-adrenoceptor agonist) does not symptomatically improve alcohol withdrawal.

Serotonin (5-HT)

- Low levels of 5-HT are associated particularly with type II alcoholism (early onset, high impulsivity, positive family history of alcoholism, male predominance):
  - increased 5-HT function may lead to craving.
- High levels of 5-HT may be associated with type I alcoholism (later onset, mixed gender, anxious):
  - increased 5-HT function may lead to anxiety.
- 5-HT is implicated in many disorders that coexist with alcoholism: depression/ suicide, anxiety disorders, bulimia nervosa.

Alcohol and other receptors

- Opioids: see 'Scientific background' above.
- Neuropeptide Y (NPY): there are many peptides that are proposed to be involved in addiction. NPY is the latest to attract attention.

Neurochemistry and neuropharmacology of treating alcohol withdrawal and dependence

Neurochemistry of alcohol withdrawal

Alcohol withdrawal is associated with:

- Increased activity in:
  - NDMA receptor
  - L-subtype of Ca^{2+} channel

$\uparrow Ca^{2+}$ influx to cell

Hyperexcitability and cell death

  - NA activity.
- Decreases in:
  - GABA function
  - Mg^{2+} inhibition of NMDA receptor
  - DA activity.

Treatment of alcohol withdrawal

- BDZs are used to increase GABA function.
- Vitamins (thiamine (B_1), B complex) are useful, as alcoholics are likely to be vitamin (especially thiamine)-deficient due to poor diet and poor absorption. Thiamine must be given parenterally if the patient is at risk of Wernicke's encephalopathy, as it is poorly absorbed orally (caution is necessary, as anaphylaxis is a rare but recognised risk). If the oral preparation is appropriate, give smaller doses more frequently to maximise absorption.

- Carbamazepine has shown efficacy, and may be an alternative if BDZs are contraindicated or ineffective.

Neurochemistry of alcohol dependence

See Fig. 7.2.

Treatment of alcohol dependence

- A variety of drugs have been used in the treatment of alcohol dependence, with limited success.
- Comorbid psychiatric disorders may require treatment, but patients should not be started on psychotropic drugs for 2–3 weeks, as symptoms may subside spontaneously with abstinence.

Some specific drugs for alcohol dependence

Disulfiram

- Disulfiram inhibits aldehyde dehydrogenase (Fig. 7.3).
- This leads to a build-up of acetaldehyde (ethanal) if alcohol is consumed, causing adverse effects:
  - nausea and vomiting
  - flushing
  - palpitations
  - headache
  - hypotension.
- Contraindications are psychosis, severe liver or cardiac disease, and epilepsy.

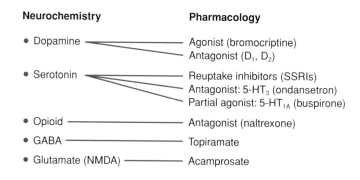

Figure 7.2 Neurochemistry related to drugs that have been used in the treatment of alcoholism. GABA, γ-aminobutyric acid; NMDA, N-methyl-D-aspartate; SSRI, selective serotonin reuptake inhibitor.

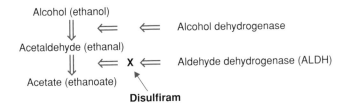

Figure 7.3 Disulfiram inhibits the metabolism of acetaldehyde to acetate.

- Supervision or witnessed consumption is associated with improved outcome.
- Disulfiram also blocks dopamine-β-hydroxylase, which may increase DA levels in the brain. It is not clear if this contributes to its efficacy.

Acamprosate

- This is a taurine derivative.
- Its exact pharmacology is still not clear, but it antagonises glutamate NMDA receptor function, possibly through an effect on α-amino-3-hydoxy-5-methyl-4-isoxazole propionate (AMPA) receptors.
- It approximately doubles abstinence rates to about 20–40% and also increases the 'time to first drink'.
- It reduces the likelihood of an episode of drinking becoming a relapse.
- Adverse effects are generally mild: gastrointestinal disturbance.
- It is contraindicated if there is severe liver damage.
- It has been described as 'anticraving', but this is contentious.
- There are no clear predictors of efficacy.
- May be neuroprotective, so consider starting during detoxification.

Naltrexone

- This is an opioid antagonist (nonselective: μ, κ, δ receptors).
- In alcohol dependence, it:
  - reduces the relapse rate
  - reduces craving.
- It is contraindicated in acute hepatitis or liver failure.

Topiramate (see also Chapter 5)

- This anticonvulsant drug has recently been reported to improve drinking behaviour (reduced drinking days, greater abstinence rates) in alcohol-dependent subjects.
- It is given when the patient is still actively drinking but in an abstinence-focused treatment plan (other trials generally give drugs when the patient is abstinent).

Treatment of comorbidity

Depression

- Depressive symptoms and disorder are common, and are as likely to precede alcohol abuse as to be a consequence of it.
- Persistent depressive symptoms following withdrawal from alcohol should be treated (see Chapter 4).
- Early trials of antidepressants in alcohol disorder and depression (tricyclic antidepressants (TCAs) and selective serotonin reuptake inhibitors (SSRIs)) did not consistently show efficacy. While depressive symptoms may improve slightly, drinking behaviour does not necessarily do so, and therefore requires treatment in its own right. There is evidence that the use of SSRIs in non-depressed type II alcohol dependence results in no improvement or maybe even worsens outcome.

Anxiety

- As with depression, anxiety may be a cause and a consequence of alcohol abuse.
- Panic attacks and generalised anxiety disorder (GAD) can emerge from alcohol dependence.
- Treatment of comorbid anxiety disorders has not been studied to the same extent as for depression.
- BDZs should rarely be used due to their addictive potential.
- Antidepressants have been shown to have some benefit in reducing panic attacks in alcoholic subjects.

Schizophrenia

- There is a fourfold increase of alcoholism in schizophrenia; it is more common than drug misuse.
- Substance misuse leads to increased family conflict (high expressed emotion) – a factor in schizophrenic relapse.
- Atypical antipsychotics may be associated with less substance misuse, including alcohol. Clozapine, in particular, has been reported to be associated with less substance misuse.

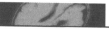 # Opiates/opioids

The term 'opiates' refers to natural substances derived from the opium poppy (e.g. morphine, codeine) and 'opioids' to all, including semisynthetic (e.g. heroin (diamorphine), dihydrocodeine (DF118)) and synthetic (e.g. methadone), compounds.

Opioids

- These act as agonists at:
  - μ (mu) receptors: analgesia, euphoria, positive reinforcement and respiratory depression. There is high-affinity binding for the endogenous ligands enkephalins and β-endorphin; morphine, codeine and methadone bind to the μ-receptor
  - κ (kappa) receptors: dysphoria, sedation and analgesia. Dynorphins are the endogenous ligands
  - δ (delta) receptors: analgesia and possibly seizures. Enkephalins are the endogenous ligands
  - σ (sigma) receptors were originally thought to be opioid receptors, but are now classified separately.
- Acute effects are miosis, euphoria, tranquillity, drowsiness, itching, nausea and respiratory depression.
- Chronic effects are anhedonia, depression, insomnia and dependence.
- The mechanism of tolerance to opioids is not well understood, with no clear changes in opioid receptor numbers reported, suggesting intracellular changes or alterations in other systems.

Opioid withdrawal

- Symptoms:
  - mydriasis, diarrhoea, dysphoria, insomnia, restlessness, 'craving'
  - associated with increased NA function: tachycardia, sweating, piloerection, rhinorrhoea, shivering.
- Opioid withdrawal is associated with increased NA function due to opioid effects in the locus ceruleus:
  - acute effects of opioids are to inhibit cyclic adenosine monophosphate (cAMP) and reduce NA neuronal firing
  - with chronic exposure, compensatory upregulation of cAMP occurs, with an increase in NA neuronal 'tone', which is revealed on withdrawal of opioids.
- Treatment:
  - opioid substitute therapy
  - symptomatic treatment for gastrointestinal disturbance, insomnia, muscle aches
  - lofexidine, an α_2-agonist, to reduce NA-related symptoms (side-effects: sedation, hypotension).

Substitute therapies in opioid addiction

- Principle: use drugs with a longer half-life than 'street' opioids (Fig. 7.4).

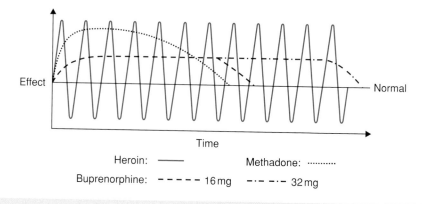

Figure 7.4 Pharmacology of opioid substitute therapy. Methadone is a relatively long-acting full agonist and buprenorphine a long-acting partial agonist, and their use avoids the 'highs' alternating with 'lows' associated with heroin (diamorphine).

Methadone

- This is a full μ-opioid agonist.
- Its half-life ($t_{1/2}$) is approximately 24 hours with regular use, but approximately 36 hours with a single dose.
- It is widely used in maintenance and detoxification.

Buprenorphine

- This is a partial agonist at the μ opioid receptor; it has a reduced risk of fatal respiratory depression.
- It is an antagonist at the κ opioid receptor, which may be why buprenorphine is less likely to cause dysphoria.
- $t_{1/2} \geqslant 24$ hours.
- The longer $t_{1/2}$ and partial agonism make the withdrawal syndrome less severe.
- It is safer than full agonists and reduces the effect of additional full (e.g. street) opiate agonists by blocking their effects (see Chapter 2 for a discussion of partial agonists).
- Due to the lower maximal effect, it can be given in larger doses, less frequently.

Naltrexone

- This is an oral nonselective opioid antagonist – blocks acute opioid effects.
- It is long-acting (the active metabolite gives an effective $t_{1/2}$ of 96 hours).
- It is used to prevent relapse in drug-free subjects.
- Good compliance and monitoring are associated with better outcome.
- The most common side-effects are gastrointestinal.

 ## Stimulants

Cocaine

- 'Crack' is the free base of cocaine, and can be smoked, inhaled or injected, giving a faster rate of onset than cocaine (snorted).
- Cocaine inhibits reuptake of DA (most important for central effects), 5-HT and NA; is a Na^+ channel blocker (local anaesthetic, cardiotoxic).
- Pharmacokinetics of delivery are important: the cocaine 'rush' intensity is due to fast uptake.
- Acute effects are euphoria (related to DA transporter blockade), confusion, psychosis, increased blood pressure/pulse (can result in stroke, seizure), formication, and then a 'crash' – see below.
- Chronic effects are paranoia, psychosis, anorexia and depression.
- There is complex adaptation to chronic use: reduced dopaminergic function, which may be partially reversible with abstinence. Reduced numbers of D_2 receptors may be associated with 'drug-liking', so low D_2 levels seen in humans may not only be a consequence of cocaine abuse.
- Withdrawal 'crash':
  - depression, anxiety, hypersomnia, anergia
  - treatment with antidepressants (desipramine) is not thought to be effective in preventing this acute 'crash'.

Pharmacotherapy for cocaine addiction under development

- Vaccines.
- Partial D_3 agonist (in animal studies, reduces response to cocaine cues).
- Drugs such as disulfiram and baclofen, and DA agonists such as bromocriptine, are also in trials.

Amfetamine

- This inhibits DA reuptake and also stimulates DA release.
- It has similar effects to cocaine.
- It is generally taken in pill form, but can be injected.

Methamfetamine

- This has a similar action to amfetamine in increasing DA through stimulating release and blocking reuptake.
- The 'high' lasts much longer, 6–8 hours, compared with the brief high from cocaine.
- It can be taken orally, snorted, smoked and injected.
- There are growing concerns about its neurotoxicity, which is likely to involve oxidative stress.

Khat (*Catha edulis*)

- This is a stimulant, with similar effects to amfetamine but much weaker.
- Leaves are chewed.
- It is currently used primarily by people from the Horn of Africa and Yemen.

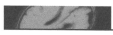 # Hallucinogens

Phencyclidine (PCP)

- This is a glutamate (NMDA) receptor antagonist.
- Acute effects:
  - delusions, paranoia, disordered thinking (schizophrenic-like), illusions/hallucinations
  - increased blood pressure/pulse.
- Chronic effects: cognitive impairment, depression and weight loss.

Ketamine

- This is another glutamate (NMDA) receptor antagonist.
- It is used as an anaesthetic agent, but is abused as a 'club drug'.
- It can be injected or snorted.
- It has similar effects to PCP: prominent dissociative effects, dream-like states and hallucinations.

Lysergic acid diethylamide (LSD)

- The primary effect is via the serotonergic system (5-HT$_{2A}$ agonist).
- Acute effects ('trip') are mood swings, delusions, synaesthesia (e.g. hearing colours), panic and increased blood pressure/pulse.
- Later effects are 'flashbacks', recurrence of unpleasant acute effects.

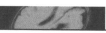 # Enactogens

The prototype is methylenedioxymethamfetamine (MDMA, Ecstasy, 'E'):

- It is stimulant/hallucinogenic, depending on the contents of the tablet.
- Derivatives: methylenedioxyamfetamine (MDA, Adam), methylenedioxyethylamfetamine (MDEA, Eve).
- These drugs are 5-HT neurotoxins (at dorsal raphe nucleus):
  - in animal studies, loss of 5-HT neurons, 5-HT transporters, decreased 5-hydroxyindoleacetic acid (5-HIAA: 5-HT metabolite) in cerebrospinal fluid

- – toxicity: MDA > MDMA > MDEA
- – neurotoxicity of MDMA in humans is not clear.
- Acute effects are empathy, increased blood pressure/pulse, dehydration, renal/heart failure, increased body temperature (greater with dancing), teeth clenching and reduced appetite.
- After-effects are midweek blues/depression and disordered sleep.
- Chronic effects are memory impairment and depression.
- Use is associated with flashbacks, psychosis, depression and anxiety.

 # Nicotine

- This is a stimulant.
- Its primary site of action is the nicotinic acetylcholine (ACh) receptor.
- It increases DA release in the NAcc by increasing firing of ventral tegmental area DA neurons.
- Tolerance is associated with receptor desensitisation and a compensatory upregulation of nicotinic receptors.
- Receptor desensitisation can lessen overnight, and hence the first cigarette of the day has the greatest effect.
- Smoking is associated with respiratory problems, many cancers and cardiovascular disease.

Treatment of nicotine addiction

- Various nicotine substitution regimens are available:
  - – the inhalator is closest in pharmacokinetic profile to smoking.
- Amfebutamone (bupropion):
  - – DA and probable NA reuptake inhibitor, which has been shown to aid smoking cessation.
- Rimonabant:
  - – cannabinoid CB_1 receptor antagonist, which has recently shown efficacy in trials.

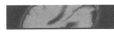 # Marijuana

Also known as cannabis, pot, weed and hash.

- The main active chemical is: Δ^9-tetrahydrocannabinol (THC), but there are up to 60, including cannabidiol, which is antipsychotic.
- The main effects of THC are mediated by binding to a G-protein-coupled receptor, known as the cannabinoid CB_1 receptor, leading to a reduction in cAMP and consequently neurotransmitter release.

- The CB_1 receptor is located on the presynaptic terminal, where it acts to inhibit release of classical neurotransmitters; it is not currently thought to be postsynaptic.
- Two putative endocannabinoid ligands for the CB_1 receptor are arachidonyl-ethanolamine (anandamide) and 2-arachidonylglycerol (2-AG).
- Anandamide has been proposed to function in a 'retrograde' manner – when a postsynaptic neuron is depolarised, anandamide is synthesised and released from the postsynaptic neuron to exert its effects through CB_1 receptors on the presynaptic neuron.
- The highest concentrations of CB_1 receptors are found in the basal ganglia and cerebellum (movement), portions of the hippocampal formation (memory). Moderately dense binding is found throughout the neocortex, particularly in the frontal, limbic and temporal lobes (cognitive and emotional functions).
- The cannabinoid CB_2 receptor is found on immune cells.
- Cannabis causes a dependence syndrome.
- Acute effects are relaxation, time confusion, feeling of 'well-being', distorted perceptions, impairment of memory, concentration and coordination, increased pulse, and anxiety,
- Chronic effects comprise the 'amotivational syndrome' – impaired attention, memory, learning, drive.
- Cannabis is psychomimetic, but this does not occur with everyone (it has recently been shown to be associated with a polymorphism of the *COMT* gene) and generally resolves. It is more controversial whether cannabis causes an enduring psychotic illness, such as schizophrenia de novo. Recent evidence has reported an increased risk of precipitating psychosis, particularly in young people. In patients with a psychotic illness, such as schizophrenia, cannabis exacerbates their psychosis and is associated with a poorer prognosis.
- Smoking is associated with respiratory problems, lung cancer and cardio-vascular disease.
- It is necessary to distinguish between smoked cannabis and the cannabis-based medicines that are showing efficacy – e.g. cannabinoid CB_1 receptor agonists in appetite stimulation, spasticity and neuropathic pain, and cannabinoid CB_1 receptor antagonists in smoking cessation and obesity.
- Evidence from animal models supports a role for the cannabinoid system in mediating effects of other drugs such as opioids and alcohol.

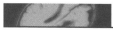γ-Hydroxybutyrate (GHB)

- GABA is a precursor of GHB.
- GHB is a depressant, and can cause respiratory arrest.
- Disinhibition, drowsiness and amnesia underlie its use as a date-rape drug.
- Its pharmacology is complex: effects are mediated through $GABA_B$ receptors and the DA, opioid and 5-HT systems.

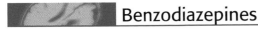

Benzodiazepines

These are discussed in Chapter 6.

Guidelines

Department of Health. Drug Misuse and Dependence – Guidelines on Clinical Management 1999 (Also known as Orange Guidelines due to colour of cover). http://www.doh.gov.uk/pub/docs/doh/dmfull.pdf

Lingford-Hughes AR, Welch S, Nutt DJ. Evidence based guidelines for the pharmacological management of substance misuse, addiction, and co-morbidity: recommendations from the British Association for Psychopharmacology. J. Psychopharmacology 2004; 18:293–335 (available at http://www.bap.org.uk) (Gives a good review of the evidence base for the treatment of addictions)

National Institute for Clinical Excellence Technology Appraisal Guidance No. 39. Guidance on the use of nicotine replacement therapy (NRT) and bupropion for smoking cessation, 2002. http://www.nice.org.uk/page.aspx?o=appraisals.completed

Scottish Intercollegiate Guidelines Network National Clinical Guideline 74. The management of harmful drinking and alcohol dependence in primary care, 2004. http://www.sign.ac.uk/guidelines/published/index.html

References

Key references

Al-Hebshi NN, Skaug N. Khat (*Catha edulis*) – an updated review. Addiction Biol 2005; 10:299–307.

Arseneault L, Cannon M, Witton J, Murray RM. Causal association between cannabis and psychosis: examination of the evidence. Br J Psychiatry 2004; 184:110–17

Foresight Brain Science Addiction and Drugs Project. A series of reviews of many aspects of addiction. http://www.foresight.gov.uk/Brain_Science_Addiction_and_Drugs/index.html

Gonzalez A, Nutt DJ. Gamma hydroxy butyrate abuse and dependency. J Psychopharmacol 2005 19:195–204

Iversen L. Cannabis and the brain. Brain 2003; 126:1252–70

Kessler RC, Crum RM, Warner LA et al. Lifetime co-occurrence of DSM-III-R alcohol abuse and dependence with other psychiatric disorders in the National Comorbidity Survey. Arch Gen Psychiatry 1997; 54:313–21

Kessler RC, McGonagle KA, Zhao S et al. Lifetime and 12–month prevalence of DSM-III-R psychiatric disorders in the United States. Arch Gen Psychiatry 1994; 51:8–19

Kreek MJ, LaForge KS, Butelman E. Pharmacotherapy of addictions. Nat Rev Drug Discov 2002; 1:710–26

Lingford-Hughes AR, Nutt D. The neurobiology of addiction and implications for treatment. Br J Psychiatry 2003; 182:97–100

Nutt DJ. Alcohol and the brain: pharmacological insights. Br J Psychiatry 1999; 175:114–19

Ward J, Hall W, Mattick RP. Role of maintenance treatment in opioid dependence. Lancet 1999; 353:221–6

Further reading

'Addiction is a brain disease, and it matters'. A series of articles in Science 1997; 278:45–70

Ashton CH. Pharmacology and effects of cannabis: a brief review. Br J Psychiatry 2000; 178:101–6 (One of a series of articles about cannabis)

Berridge KC, Robinson TE. What is the role of dopamine in reward: hedonic impact, reward learning or incentive salience? Brain Res Rev 1998; 28:309–69

Di Chiara G. A motivational learning hypothesis of the role of mesolimbic dopamine in compulsive drug use. J Psychopharmacol 1998; 12:54–67

Dual Diagnosis. A series of articles in Biol Psychiatry 2004; 56:703–818

Garbutt JC, West SL, Carey TS, Lohr KN, Crews FT. Pharmacological treatment of alcohol dependence: a review of the evidence. JAMA 1999; 281:1318–25

Kalivas PW, Volkow ND. The neural basis of addiction: a pathology of motivation and choice Am J Psychiatry 2005: 162:1403–13

Koob GF, Ahmed SH, Boutrel B et al. Neurobiological mechanisms in the transition from drug use to drug dependence. Neurosci Biobehav Rev 2004: 27:739–49

Soyka M. Alcoholism and schizophrenia. Addiction 2000; 95:1613–18

Volkow ND, Fowler JS, Wang GJ. The addicted human brain viewed in the light of imaging studies: brain circuits and treatment strategies. Neuropharmacology 2004; 47:3–13.

Volkow ND, Li TK. Drugs and alcohol: treating and preventing abuse, addiction and their medical consequences. Pharmacol Ther 2005; 108:3–17

Ziedonis DM, Smelson D, Rosenthal RN et al. Improving the care of individuals with schizophrenia and substance use disorders: consensus recommendations. J Psychiatr Pract 2005; 11:315–39

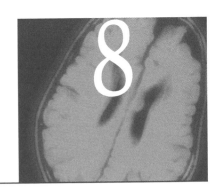

Drugs for dementia

N Harry P Allen

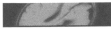 ## Types of dementia

- Two main types of symptoms require treatment in the dementias:
  - cognitive deficits (ranging from mild to severe)
  - noncognitive features (behavioural and psychiatric symptoms of dementia (BPSD), consisting of affective, psychotic and behavioural disturbances).
- Types of dementia relevant to treatment:
  - Alzheimer's disease (AD)
  - dementia with Lewy bodies (DLB) (commonly with motor features of Parkinson's disease)
  - vascular dementia (multi-infarct dementia, small-vessel dementia, infarcts of strategic areas).

 ## History

- The cholinergic hypothesis of AD led to initial studies of the acetylcholine (ACh) precursors lecithin and choline, with little benefit.
- Cholinesterase inhibitors (also called anticholinesterases):
  - tetrahydroaminoacridine (tacrine, THA) was originally developed as an antiseptic in the 1940s and was then used as a respiratory stimulant to reverse anaesthesia in the UK and Australia. It was first tested in AD in the 1980s; it is licensed in the USA
  - donepezil, rivastigmine and galantamine are licensed in the UK
  - these are the subject of a Clinical Practice Guideline from the UK National Institute for Clinical Excellence (NICE) in 2001. Reappraisal second draft guideline as at February 2006 proposes limiting treatment with cholinesterase inhibitors to patients with moderately severe dementia only, and excludes mildly impaired patients from treatment (which is new) and continues to exclude severely impaired patients from treatment. The draft guideline also proposes that memantine not be used unless in the setting of a clinical trial.

▓ Glutamate antagonist (memantine):
- this was introduced in Germany in 1982 for organic brain syndromes
- it was licensed in Europe in 2002 for AD.

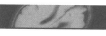 Scientific background

Alzheimer's disease

Figure 8.1 outlines risk factors, pathology and treatment targets in AD.

Targets for drug intervention

▓ There is potential for future intervention at the level of genes, nerve growth factors and neuropathological changes.

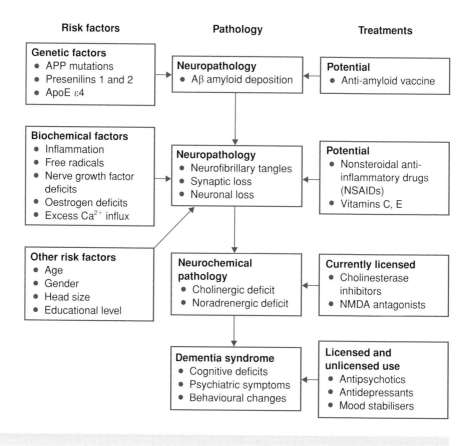

Figure 8.1   Risk factors, pathology and treatment of Alzheimer's disease.

- Inflammation/neuroprotection:
    - chronic nonsteroidal anti-inflammatory drugs (NSAIDs) decrease the risk of AD by two to four times
    - oestrogen delays the onset of AD. Possible mechanisms include reversal of glucocorticoid damage, increased cerebral blood flow, prevention of neuronal atrophy, and synergistic action with nerve growth factors
    - regular vitamin supplements (C or E) in the elderly are associated with a lower risk of developing AD, possibly by reducing oxidative stress
    - amyloid is a potential target, specifically the development of the Aβ peptide fragment from amyloid precursor protein (APP). Secretase inhibitors to promote the production of the non-amyloidogenic α-fragment from APP are under development.
- For neurochemistry, see below.

Cholinergic hypothesis of AD

Figure 8.2 outlines the main metabolic pathways of ACh (see also Chapter 1).

- Antimuscarinic drugs (e.g. scopolamine) induce memory deficits and confusion in normal subjects.

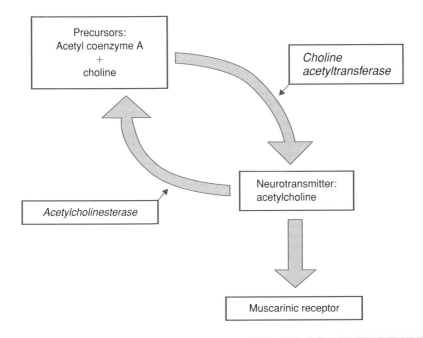

Figure 8.2 The metabolic pathway of acetylcholine production and removal (see also Chapter 1).

- In AD:
    - there is substantial loss of cholinergic neurons in the nucleus basalis (of Meynert), the origin of the cholinergic pathway projecting to all cortical areas and part of the thalamus
    - postmortem estimates of cholinergic function correlate with mental test scores and amyloid plaque counts
    - there is reduced choline acetyltransferase (ChAT), choline uptake and ACh release in neocortex.
- Two cholinesterases are present – acetylcholinesterase (AChE) and butyryl-cholinesterase (BuChE, previously known as pseudocholinesterase):
    - AChE is found in cholinergic synapses in the central nervous system (CNS) and periphery
    - BuChE is synthesised in the liver and secreted into plasma. It is also present in glial cells. Inhibition may lead to unwanted peripheral side-effects.

Monoamine deficits in AD

These may account for behavioural changes in AD.

- Noradrenaline (NA) is reduced especially in temporal cortex: loss of noradren-ergic neurons and monoamine oxidase (MAO) are associated with depressive symptoms, and may also relate to deficits in attention. Relative preservation of NA activity has been associated with delusions.
- Loss of serotonin (5-HT) function is present in later stages: may relate to aggression, mood change.
- Dopamine (DA), γ-aminobutyric acid (GABA) and somatostatin concentrations are not significantly changed.

Mechanism of neuronal damage in AD

There are probably several mechanisms for neuronal damage in AD:
- Influx of Ca^{2+} ions facilitated by glutamate causes neuronal death:
    - prevention or reduction of this influx may be neuroprotective
    - blockade of the glutamate N-methyl-D-aspartate (NMDA) receptor may be one way to achieve this.

Dementia with Lewy bodies

- The greater cholinergic impairment than in AD is correlated with visual hallucinations.
- There is relative preservation of muscarinic M_1 receptors.
- DLB may respond to procholinergic treatment. Noncognitive symptoms (especially visual hallucinations) may respond better than cognitive symptoms.

Vascular dementia

- Vascular pathology is the target for treatment.
- Control of hypertension and diabetes is effective in prevention.

 ## Assessment of outcome in clinical trials

Assessment is difficult and interpretation may be problematic; prevention of deterioration is important, as well as improvement.

Table 8.1 outlines the domains of assessment and the major assessment rating scales.

 ## Drug treatment

- Genetic considerations:
  - effectiveness of cholinesterases is reduced in ApoE ε4 carriers
  - ApoE ε4 carriers may respond better to noncholinergic treatments, e.g. the MAO-B inhibitor selegiline.
- Vaccines:
  - vaccines against aggregated Aβ have been tested. Encephalitis has developed in test subjects
  - a future refinement is the development of vaccine against the N-terminal end of amyloid, with reduction in associated side-effects.
- Future possibilities include the development of secretase inhibitors.

Cholinergic precursors

- Precursor loading with choline or lecithin.
- Ineffective.
- Side-effect of rotting fish smell with choline.

Cholinesterase inhibitors

General issues

- There is potentiation of remaining cholinergic function, so the potential benefit is related to the amount of remaining function.
- They are most effective in the early stages of dementia, but efficacy is lost as dementia progresses (however, note the NICE reappraisal in mild AD: Table 8.2).
- Gastrointestinal side-effects are dose-related.
- Rarer adverse effects are stomach ulcers, sinoatrial block and atrioventricular block, seizures, and transient ischaemic attacks.

> **Table 8.1** Domains and rating scales in clinical trials of dementia
>
> **Cognitive performance**
> - Alzheimer's Disease Assessment Scale (ADAS-cog): tests multiple areas of cognitive decline. Error score 0–70. Low score = high performance. Usually a primary outcome variable
> - Mini-mental State Examination (MMSE): screening instrument briefly tests several areas of cognition, but not in depth. Score 0 (low performance) to 30 (high performance)
> - Numerous others, e.g. Abbreviated Mental Test Score (AMTS)
>
> **Global outcome measures**
> - Clinicians Interview Based Impression of Change (CIBIC): interview-based assessment of global functioning. Score 1 (very much improved) to 7 (very much worse). CIBIC-plus includes interview with carer. Usually a primary outcome variable
> - Clinical Dementia Rating (CDR): six domains rating deterioration in ability. Score 0 to 3 (severe)
>
> **Functional ability/activities of daily living (ADL)**
> - Instrumental Activities of Daily Living (IADL): ability on household tasks, slightly adjusted for gender
> - Interview for Deterioration in Daily Living in Dementia (IDDD): deterioration in simple and more complex areas of daily living activity
>
> **Behaviour and mood**
> - Neuropsychiatric Inventory (NPI): psychiatric and behavioural changes in 12 domains
> - Manchester and Oxford Universities Scale for the Psychopathological Assessment of Dementia (MOUSEPAD): semistructured interview of psychopathological and behavioural changes. Rates frequency only

- Interactions:
  - cholinesterase inhibitors are antagonised by procainamide, quinidine, aminoglycosides and antimuscarinic drugs
  - drugs used in anaesthesia: depolarising muscle relaxants (e.g. suxamethonium) may be potentiated; nondepolarising muscle relaxants (e.g. pancuronium) may be antagonised
  - galantamine metabolism is reduced by some cytochrome P450 (CYP450) inhibitors (e.g. paroxetine, ketoconazole, erythromycin), leading to increased plasma concentrations.

Prescribing issues

Funding/implementation issues have led to variable availability in the UK. This is the subject of a national guideline from NICE, requiring availability of licensed cholinesterase inhibitors (donepezil, rivastigmine, galantamine) subject to specific requirements. A reappraisal is likely to further restrict use to moderate AD only (Table 8.2).

Table 8.2   Summary of NICE guidance for the use of drug treatment for Alzheimer's disease (AD)

2001 guidance
- Diagnosis of AD made in specialist clinic according to standard diagnostic criteria
- Likelihood of compliance assessed
- Tests required of cognitive, global and behavioural functioning and ADL before drug prescription
- Initiation and maintenance prescription only if MMSE >12
- Initial prescription only by specialists, and transfer to general practitioners only recommended if agreed shared care protocol and agreed endpoints
- Reassessment of progress after 2–4 months, and drug continued only if global improvement together with cognitive improvement or lack of decline
- Reassessment every 6 months if drug continued

2006 reappraisal consultation (final decision expected mid-2006)
- Proposed restriction to MMSE between 10–20, i.e. not in mild or severe AD (poor evidence of clinically significant benefit)
- Guidance extended to memantine (likely to be recommended only in context of a clinical trial)

ADL, Activities of Daily Living; MMSE, Mini-Mental State Examination.

Tacrine (tetrahydroaminoacridine, THA), velnacrine

- These are reversible cholinesterase inhibitors; velnacrine is a derivative of THA.
- Several studies have reported that THA significantly improves ADAS-cog, CIBIC and MMSE scores.
- Hepatic toxicity is dose-dependent.
- THA is licensed in the USA and France, but not in the UK. There is no licence for velnacrine.

Metrifonate

- This was originally developed to treat parasitic worms (schistosomiasis).
- Modest improvements have been found in ADAS-cog and CIBIC. There are inconsistent results with secondary variables.
- It is generally well tolerated; side-effects are mainly gastrointestinal and muscle weakness.
- It is not licensed.

Donepezil

- This piperidine derivative is a reversible cholinesterase inhibitor with high specificity for AChE over BuChE (this may reduce peripheral side-effects).

- The long elimination half-life (70–80 hours) allows once-daily dosage.
- It is metabolised by the liver, and is not associated with hepatic toxicity.
- *Efficacy*: there have been eight randomised controlled trials (RCTs) and a number of systematic reviews:
  - improved CIBIC (cf. decline with placebo)
  - dose-response on ADAS-cog up to 10 mg/day
  - improvements over baseline decline with time as the disease progresses
  - generally no significant improvement in quality of life (QoL) measures.
- It is licensed in the UK, and is awaiting NICE re-evaluation (Table 8.2).

Rivastigmine

- This carbamate derivative is a reversible cholinesterase inhibitor.
- It is rapidly absorbed, and is best taken with food to improve tolerability.
- The short elimination half-life (<2 hours) necessitates twice-daily dosage.
- It is metabolised by cholinesterases, predominantly in the liver.
- *Efficacy*: there have been seven RCTs and a number of systematic reviews:
  - improved global outcome measures in some individual studies compared with placebo (but not robust in pooled data)
  - inconsistent effect on cognitive measures, which appears effective at higher doses only
  - significant improvement in QoL measures in only one trial.
- It is licensed in the UK, and is awaiting NICE re-evaluation (Table 8.2).

Galantamine

- This tertiary alkaloid is a reversible cholinesterase inhibitor; it also potentiates the action of ACh at nicotinic receptors.
- It is well absorbed orally, with low protein binding.
- The short elimination half-life (7 hours) necessitates twice-daily dosage. A slow-release preparation is available, with once-a-day dosing.
- It is metabolised by CYP450 2D6 and 3A4, with no significant active metabolites.
- *Efficacy*: there have been six RCTs and three systematic reviews:
  - improved CIBIC compared with placebo (statistically significant only at higher doses)
  - dose-response improvements in ADAS-cog scores
  - improvements in ADL at 6 months
  - improvements in QoL measures at 6 months.
- It is licensed in the UK, and is awaiting NICE re-evaluation (Table 8.2).

Glutamate antagonist

Memantine

- This is a low- to moderate-affinity noncompetitive NMDA antagonist.
- The elimination half-life is 60–80 hours.

- *Efficacy:* There is limited trial evidence from two RCTs in moderate to severe AD:
  - significant effects in cognition and ADL compared with placebo
  - benefits in combination with donepezil in cognition and ADL.
- Side-effects are hallucinations and confusion.
- It is awaiting NICE evaluation (expected 2006: the consultation document indicates no endorsement; see Table 8.2); prescribing in the UK is currently patchy as a result.

Nootropics

- Examples are piracetam, pramiracetam and oxiracetam.
- They improve memory in animal models by an unknown mechanism, possibly metabolic enhancement.
- There is limited evidence of improvement in patients with dementia.

Hormone replacement therapy (HRT)

- Potential benefits are suggested by epidemiological data.
- Meta-analysis of five trials showed a limited positive effect from low-dose replacement (1.3 MMSE point gain after 2 months).
- Reduction in behavioural and psychiatric symptoms of dementia has also been reported with HRT.
- Controlled trials are ongoing.
- The risk–benefit ratio needs evaluation in light of current concerns about the increased risk of breast cancer and stroke with long-term HRT.

Drugs for vascular dementia

- Salicylate inhibits platelet cyclo-oxygenase and reduces platelet stickiness. Aspirin has been shown to improve cognition.
- Cholinesterase inhibitors:
  - showed modest improvements in a 6-month controlled trial
  - are as well tolerated in vascular dementia as in AD
  - have a possible use in combination with memantine in the future.
- Ca^{2+} antagonists: nimodipine. The final common pathway in cell death is an increase in intracellular Ca^{2+}. These have potential use in small-vessel dementia.
- Agents that improve red blood cell deformability and thereby enhance oxygen delivery (e.g. pentoxyphylline) may be effective in large-vessel dementia.
- Propentofylline, a xanthine derivative, protects against cell damage by increasing extracellular adenosine. This reduces the damaging activation of microglia. Preliminary results promising.
- Vasodilators (e.g. cyclandelate, papaverine, cinnarizine) are ineffective.

- Ergot derivatives: mechanism is unknown. They show very modest improvements compared with placebo.
- *Ginkgo biloba* has been reported to decrease platelet aggregation and blood viscosity through an unknown mechanism. It is effective in controlled studies. Side-effects include subarachnoid or subdural haemorrhage.

Drugs for dementia with Lewy bodies

- There is significant cholinergic deficit in this condition.
- Cholinesterase inhibitors appear effective as for AD, but are outside the current UK licence.

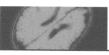

Treatment of behavioural and psychiatric symptoms of dementia (BPSD)

Principles

- Careful definition of symptoms is necessary, with elimination/treatment of physical causes (e.g. infections, cardiovascular disease, constipation).
- Optimise the personal and physical environment, consider psychosocial factors and educate carers.
- Avoid/minimise drug causes, e.g. antimuscarinic drugs (worsen cognition), anti-adrenergic drugs (postural hypotension) and drugs with long elimination half-life.

Depressive symptoms/disorders

- These are common but underdiagnosed and undertreated.
- There have been few treatment studies: antidepressants may be useful. Selective serotonin reuptake inhibitors (SSRIs) are probably preferred over older tricyclic antidepressants (TCAs).
- Review and consider stopping antidepressant after 6–12 months; depression often goes as dementia progresses.

Psychotic symptoms

- These are more common in AD than in vascular dementia.
- Typical antipsychotics have been the traditional treatment, with no evidence that any one is more effective than another. Extrapyramidal side-effects (EPSEs) occur especially in DLB.
- Atypical antipsychotics have increasingly been used: they produce fewer EPSEs and less cognitive impairment than typicals. Their long-term safety is not proven.

- – in 2004, the Committee on Safety of Medicines (CSM) in the UK issued a warning of increased risk of cerebrovascular adverse events in elderly patients taking olanzapine and risperidone (approximately 3% vs 1% over 12 weeks). The risk is especially raised in those with pre-existing cerebrovascular disease
- – the mechanism, and risk with other antipsychotics, is unclear, but there is increasing evidence that typical antipsychotics have the same stroke risk as atypicals.
- ▥ Plan to stop treatment after 3–9 months, as psychosis often goes as dementia progresses.

Agitation/aggression

- ▥ Antipsychotic drugs are the mainstay of treatment (see the previous section for issues in prescribing).
- ▥ CSM (2004) advised that olanzapine and risperidone should not be used for behavioural symptoms in dementia because of risk of stroke, but it is not clear that other antipsychotics are any better. The Royal College of Psychiatrists (2005) has issued advice on prescribing in this situation.

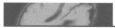 **Guidelines**

National Institute for Clinical Excellence Technology Appraisal Guidance No. 19. Guidance on the use of donepezil, rivastigmine and galantamine for the treatment of Alzheimer's disease, 2001. http://www.nice.org.uk/page.aspx?o=appraisals.completed (Re-evaluation underway and results expected 2006; includes review of evidence of drug efficacy)
Royal College of Psychiatrists Faculty for the Psychiatry of Old Age. Atypical antipsychotic and behavioural and psychiatric symptoms of dementia: prescribing update for old age psychiatrists, 2005. http://www.rcpsych.ac.uk/college/faculty/oap/BPSD.pdf

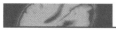 **References**

Key references

Bowen DM, Smith CB, White P, Davidson AN. Neurotransmitter-related enzymes and indices of hypoxia in senile dementia and other abiotrophies. Brain 1976; 99:459–96
Perry EK, Tomlinson BE, Blessed G et al. Correlation of cholinergic abnormalities with senile plaques and mental test scores in senile dementia. BMJ 1978; ii:1457–9
Schneider LS, Pollock VE, Lyness SA. A meta-analysis of controlled trials of neuroleptic treatment in dementia. J Am Geriatr Soc 1990; 38:553–63.
Wolfson C, Moride Y, Perrault A et al. Drug Treatments for Alzheimer's Disease. 1. Comparative Analysis of Clinical Trials. Ottawa: Canadian Coordinating Office for Health Technology Assessment (CCOHTA), 2000

Further reading

Allen NHP, Burns AB. The non-cognitive features of dementia. Rev Clin Ger 1995; 5:57–75

Alzheimer A. On certain peculiar disease of old age. Hist Psychiatry 1991; ii:71–101

Bryson HM, Benfield P. Donepezil. Drugs Aging 1997; 10:234–9.

Clegg A, Bryant J, Nicholson T et al. Clinical and cost-effectiveness of donepezil, rivastigmine and galantamine for Alzheimer's disease. Health Technology Assessment Report on Behalf of the National Institute for Clinical Excellence, 2000. http://www.nice.org.uk

Committee on Safety of Medicines. Atypical antipsychotic drugs and stroke, 2004. http://www.mhra.gov.uk/home/groups/pl-p/documents/drugsafetymessage/con019488.pdf

Forette F, Seux M-L, Staessen JA et al. Prevention of dementia in randomised double-blind placebo-controlled systolic hypertension in Europe (Syst-Eur) trial. Lancet 1998; 351: 1347–51

Morris MC, Beckett LA, Scherr PA et al. Vitamin E and vitamin C supplement use and risk of incident Alzheimer disease. Alzheimer Dis Assoc Disord 1998; 12:121–6

O'Brien J, Ames D, Burns A (eds). Dementia, 2nd edn. Oxford: Arnold, 2000

Scott LJ, Goa KL. Galantamine. Drugs Aging 2000; 60:1095–122

Spencer CM, Noble S. Rivastigmine. Drugs Aging 1998; 13:391–411

Website: http://www.alzheimers.org.uk/Facts_about_dementia/index.htm

Drugs for personality disorders and rapid tranquillisation

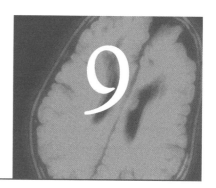

Ian C Reid and Ian M Anderson

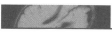 ## Background

- The pharmacological treatment of personality disorders is a relatively poorly researched and evidenced field.
- Clinical trials to date have, in general, studied few patients (numbers in the region of 10–30 per group per trial), have had short durations of treatment (weeks), have tended to use inconsistent outcome measures, and have tended to have high dropout rates.
- A recently published Cochrane review found only 10 short randomised controlled trials (RCTs) with data that could be entered into a meta-analysis.
- In the last few years, this situation has been improving, particularly in North America. Nonetheless, much of the work to date has focused on females with borderline personality disorder.

Classification of personality disorder

- The DSM-IV classification system is the most widely used classification system in clinical research with personality disordered subjects.
- Disorders are grouped into three clusters (A, B and C (Table 9.1) on Axis II of the diagnostic schedule.
- There are significant problems with the classification system for clinical and basic researchers:
  - the diagnostic categories have overlapping features: individuals are commonly comorbid for more than one Axis II disorder, and comorbidity with Axis I disorders is also common
  - these two factors mean that clinical trials, even when utilising careful diagnostic criteria, necessarily study heterogeneous populations of patients
  - an aspect of the core definition of personality disorder (in particular, the issue of persistence) has been challenged. A recent long-term follow-up study found that outcome in borderline personality disorder is far better than previously realised.

Table 9.1   Diagnostic criteria and types of personality disorder (based on DSM-IV)

Diagnosis

An enduring pattern of inner experience and behaviour that deviates markedly from the expectations of the individual's culture, with abnormalities in at least two of the following areas: cognition, affectivity (emotional responsivity), interpersonal functioning, impulse control.

The pattern is inflexible and pervasive, stable, and of long duration, starting in adolescence or early adulthood, and leads to clinically significant distress or impairment in functioning.

It is not better accounted for by another mental or physical disorder or the physiological effects of a substance.

Types

Cluster A: Odd–eccentric personality disorders
   Paranoid
   Schizoid
   Schizotypal
Cluster B: Dramatic–emotional–erratic personality disorders
   Antisocial
   Borderline
   Histrionic
   Narcissistic
Cluster C: Anxious–fearful personality disorders
   Avoidant
   Dependent
   Obsessive–compulsive

■   Thus, heterogeneity and comorbidity among clinical samples, and the poor predictive validity of our clinical constructs, considerably hamper neurobiological and pharmacological research.

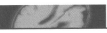 Theoretical issues

■   The aetiology of the personality disorders is complex, encompassing genetic, biological and environmental/social factors.
■   For example, in borderline personality disorder:
   –   the estimated monozygotic-to-dizygotic concordance ratio is as high as 5 : 1 (i.e. similar in magnitude to schizophrenia) in some twin studies
   –   recent neuroimaging studies suggest functional and structural changes in frontal and temporal lobes
   –   there is a clear association with early childhood trauma.
■   Attempts have been made to link dimensions of normal and abnormal personality to specific neurotransmitter systems in order to provide a rationale for

pharmacotherapy. Cloninger and colleagues (1993) proposed a psychobiology of temperament (inherited tendencies) and character (environmentally acquired personality features) that relates:

- *novelty seeking* (inherited tendency to exploratory activity and intense excitement in response to novel stimuli) to dopamine (DA) function
- *harm avoidance* (inherited tendency to respond intensely to aversive stimuli, and to avoid punishment, novelty and non-reward) to serotonin (5-HT) function
- *reward dependence* (inherited tendency to respond intensely to reward and maintenance of rewarded behaviour) to noradrenaline (NA) function.

- Unfortunately, this neat notion has limited empirical support. It has nonetheless provided a useful framework and stimulus for research, and a spur to thinking about personality disorder beyond a purely descriptive classification.
- Pharmacotherapy of a personality disordered subject can be thought of as being based on three main rationales:
  - a presumed 'spectrum' with an equivalent Axis I disorder (e.g antipsychotics for the paranoid personality disorder–schizophrenia spectrum; anxiolytics and SSRIs for the avoidant personality disorder–anxiety disorder spectrum)
  - symptom relief, rather than treatment of the core disorder: it is notable, for example, that in some studies of borderline personality disorder, antipsychotics may have beneficial effects that extend beyond 'psychosis-like symptoms' to impact on mood and self harm
  - theoretical grounds (e.g. treatment of presumed low-5-HT conditions such as aggression/impulsivity/suicidality with selective serotonin reuptake inhibitors (SSRIs) based on the putative neurochemistry of Cloninger's temperamental types).

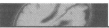 # Treatment of personality disorder

Psychological treatment

- Psychological approaches provide the mainstay for the treatment of personality disorder.
- Systematic reviews emphasise the use of dynamic psychotherapy, cognitive therapy, cognitive analytic therapy, dialectical behaviour therapy (DBT) and therapeutic community treatments, and the evidence base for the efficacy (if not yet the generalisability) of such treatments is growing.

Pharmacological treatment

- The majority of trials to date have been conducted with patients suffering from borderline personality disorder:

- the evidence base is growing, with larger, higher-quality, randomised and blinded trials being initiated. Dropout rates are falling and, diagnostic fidelity is improving
- however, there remains a lack of consensus on outcome measures and an over-reliance on subscale analysis.
- Pharmacological approaches centre on three main classes of drugs: antidepressants, antipsychotics and 'mood stabilisers'.

Antipsychotics

- This is probably the most widely used drug category in the treatment of personality disorder.
- Trials vary in size and quality (many are 'open-label') – dropout rates are often high (50%).
- Haloperidol, olanzapine, risperidone and quetiapine have all been suggested to have an impact on a range of symptoms, including depression, interpersonal sensitivity, psychoticism and hostility.
- Haloperidol may be better than antidepressants for hostility and psychoticism.
- Case reports suggest that clozapine may reduce rates of self-harm.
- There is some evidence that the addition of antipsychotics (e.g. olanzapine) may improve outcomes in patients receiving psychotherapy (e.g. DBT).

Antidepressants

- Tricyclic antidepressants (TCAs), venlafaxine, SSRIs and monoamine oxidase inhibitors (MAOIs) have all been evaluated, with some promising results.
- SSRIs:
  - it has been suggested that these may in particular reduce impulsiveness, self-harm and anger
  - however, it is difficult to distinguish effects on comorbid mood disorder from impact on 'core' personality disorder
  - trials combining SSRIs with psychotherapy have yielded inconsistent results
  - limited trial evidence suggests a possible value in combining antidepressants and antipsychotics (this is common in clinical practice).

'Mood stabilisers' (lithium and anticonvulsants)

- Lithium, carbamazepine, lamotrigine, topiramate, valproate and phenytoin have all been evaluated to some extent.
- Trials have been short: 8–12 weeks.
- Sample size has mostly been small: 30–50 subjects.
- Significant reductions in depression, impulsivity and anger expression have been reported, but results are inconsistent.

Benzodiazepines (BDZs)

- These are often used (or end up being used for a variety of reasons, including 'self-prescription') in patients with personality disorder.
- There is no substantial evidence that this class of drugs is of value, and there is a theoretical risk of disinhibition.
- The risks of dependence may be greater among these patients.
- Therefore the usual considerations regarding BDZs apply, related to the possibility of tolerance, the risk of dose escalation, and limiting dose and length of use (see Chapter 6).

Principles of drug therapy

- In treating individuals with personality disorder, the following factors need to be considered (based on principles of good clinical practice in the absence of evidence):
  - give a detailed explanation of any proposed pharmacotherapy: discuss side-effects and agree aims and desired outcomes with the patient
  - in particular, specify a few target symptoms and agree how to evaluate them (e.g. a simple rating scale)
  - do not allow the number of drugs to accumulate: evaluate one agent at a time
  - make a joint plan, specifying agent and duration of trial; plan the review frequency; outline the next steps if the outcome is unsatisfactory
  - do not be afraid to discontinue medications that have been tried at a satisfactory dose for a reasonable length of time but without *any* sign of benefit (6–8 weeks is a good rule of thumb). Gradually reduce the doses of drugs being discontinued
  - consider potential toxicity and limit prescription size in self-harming patients.

 # Rapid tranquillisation

- The use of pharmacotherapy to induce rapid tranquillisation (RT) in acutely disturbed patients is considered briefly here because, as with the treatment of personality-disordered subjects, it is targeted principally at symptoms and behaviour rather than directly at an underlying disorder.
- The National Institute for Clinical Excellence (NICE, 2005) have published comprehensive guidelines on the short-term management of violence, covering a wide range of issues (Table 9.2).

Environmental and psychological management

- It is important to stress that the first steps in dealing with acute behavioural disturbance do not involve drugs.

Table 9.2 Summary of topics covered in NICE (2005) guidance on the short-term management of violence

- Environment, organisation and alarm systems
- Prediction of violence (antecedents, warning signs and risk assessment)
- Staff training
- Service user perspectives, including those relating to ethnicity, gender and other special concerns
- Searching of patients, their belongings and environment
- Use of de-escalation techniques
- Appropriate and effective observation
- Use of physical intervention
- Use of seclusion
- Rapid tranquillisation
- Post-incident reviews
- Specific issues for emergency departments

- The emphasis should be on efforts to 'talk down' the patient, while paying commonsense attention to environmental issues and the safety and dignity of the patient, clinical staff and others.
- Even in the most urgent of situations, it is important to give due consideration to assessment: diagnostic, interpersonal and sustaining factors are all relevant.
- Adequate training of all staff is necessary.

Pharmacological management

General considerations

- The pharmacological management of violence/behavioural emergencies (RT) is targeted at symptoms/behaviour, not the underlying disorder. However, for the majority of cases in psychiatric services, a psychotic disorder will be present and antipsychotics may be appropriate for the acute situation as well as the underlying disorder.
- Recent emphasis on the desired outcome of RT is the recipient being 'calm and conscious' rather than 'asleep'.
- RT must always be in the context of psychological and environmental management, and is not a substitute for it.
- RT is not without risk, whatever the agent used, and safety is a primary consideration. However, not adequately treating behavioural disturbance is also risky – it is the balance of risks that needs to be considered.
- If general non-pharmacological measures are ineffective or inappropriate then oral administration is the first route of choice. Only if this proves impractical should parenteral administration be considered.

▦ Escalating situations and past history should guide the timing of RT: early oral administration may prevent the need for later parenteral drugs.

▦ A clear treatment plan should be recorded, including timing and dose of subsequent drug administration.

▦ The management plan should be reviewed regularly, and at least every 24 hours.

Choice of drugs for rapid tranquillisation

▦ The choice of agent(s) centres on antipsychotics, BDZs or both (see Table 9.3 for drugs commonly used in RT and comments on individual drugs).

▦ Liquid preparations or disintegrating tablets are useful to ensure absorption when drugs are given orally.

▦ An antipsychotic is a reasonable choice if it is also an appropriate treatment for the underlying disorder; otherwise lorazepam should be considered.

▦ Combined haloperidol plus lorazepam is commonly used clinically in more severe situations, but there is little evidence for benefit over either given individually.

▦ Evidence:
  - overall, there is a lack of good-quality trial evidence for the efficacy and safety of drugs used in RT
  - a Cochrane review comparing BDZ, antipsychotics and the combination found no difference between groups (however, there was insufficient evidence to be confident that differences did not exist)
  - in the two largest RCTs to date (500 patients altogether), both intramuscular haloperidol plus promethazine and intramuscular BDZs (lorazepam or midazolam) were effective, with midazolam being more sedative than the combination in one study and lorazepam less sedative in the other. Serious adverse events were rare.

▦ Parenteral administration:
  - guidelines on parenteral administration abound. A recent review concluded that among the antipsychotics, intramuscular haloperidol, chlorpromazine and zuclopenthixol acetate are all associated with potentially serious side-effects, and that parenteral atypical formulations (e.g. olanzapine, ziprasidone) may prove promising alternatives
  - particular attention should be drawn to cardiac and extrapyramidal side-effects as important limitations, particularly if antipsychotic drugs are given intravenously (it is debatable whether this is ever warranted)
  - the main concern with parenteral BDZs is respiratory depression (especially if other sedative drugs have been taken). However, overall, intramuscular lorazepam appears to be the safest and most practical first-line current option. BDZ-induced disinhibition appears unlikely in the acute situation
  - parenteral treatment should only be used if it is possible to undertake careful observation and monitoring, there are resuscitation facilities, and flumazenil (BDZ antagonist) is available if lorazepam is used

Table 9.3 Drugs in current use for rapid tranquillisation

Drug	Oral[a]	Parenteral[a]	Comments and precautions
Antipsychotics			
Chlorpromazine	50–200 mg (1 g)	Do not use	Not recommended by NICE (2005) because of cardiac concerns
Haloperidol	5–20 mg (30 mg)	5–18 mg (18 mg)	Preferred initial antipsychotic in severe disturbance; use with anticholinergic. Can be combined with lorazepam if necessary
Olanzapine	5–20 mg (20 mg)	5–10 mg (20 mg) IM only	Do not give IM within 1 hour of intramuscular lorazepam, because of concerns about cardiorespiratory depression. Not recommended in dementia (see Chapter 8)
Risperidone	2–4 mg (16 mg)	Not available	Not recommended in dementia (see Chapter 8)
Zuclopenthixol acetate (Acuphase)	Not applicable	50–150 mg (150 mg) IM only	Do not use in antipsychotic-naive patients; only use if repeated IM injection/prolonged disturbance/good previous response. Not routinely recommended by NICE (2005)
Benzodiazepines[b]			
Diazepam	5–10 mg (30 mg)	Do not use IM	Not routinely recommended
Lorazepam	1–4 mg (16 mg)	1–4 mg (16 mg)	Dilute with equal volume of sterile saline or water. Do not mix in same syringe as antipsychotic
Others			
Promethazine	25–50 mg (100 mg)	25–50 mg (100 mg)	Antihistamine. Used safely with haloperidol in large RCTs. Not recommended by NICE (2005)
Paraldehyde	Not applicable	5–10 mL (20 mL) IM only	Only exceptional use. Avoid more than brief contact with plastic syringe (dissolves plastic)

[a] Single dose, with 24-hour maximum dose in parentheses. Doses are illustrative – consult the British National Formulary and NICE/local guidelines in clinical situations.
[b] Midazolam (used in premedication and anaesthesia) was used intramuscularly in the largest RCT of rapid tranquillisation, but is not included in this table because of its short half-life (2–3 hours) and lack of general clinical experience.
IM, intramuscular; RCT, randomised controlled trial.

- NICE guidance (2005) recommends only haloperidol, olanzapine and lorazepam for intramuscular use in RT (but note the RCT evidence with promethazine).
- It is not uncommon for high doses of drugs to be used knowingly or inadvertently. When it is necessary to use high doses, consult guidance on high-dose antipsychotic prescribing (e.g. Royal College of Psychiatrists consensus statement).
- The management of behavioural disturbance extends beyond the acute phase. Planning ongoing pharmacology management is important, as is addressing the impact on the patient (and sometimes staff).

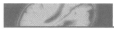 ## Guidelines

National Institute for Clinical Excellence Clinical Guideline 25. Violence – The short-term management of disturbed/violent behaviour in in-patient psychiatric settings and emergency departments, 2005. http://www.nice.org.uk/page.aspx?o= guidelines.completed

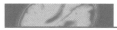 ## References

Key references

Binks CA, Fenton M, McCarthy L et al. Pharmacological interventions for people with border-line personality disorder. Cochrane Database Syst Rev 2006, (1):CD005653.

Bateman AW, Tyrer P. Personality disorder: No longer a diagnosis of exclusion: policy implementation guidance for the development of services for people with personality disorder. Department of Health, 2003. http://www.publications.doh.gov.uk/mentalhealth/personality disorder.htm

Tyrer P, Bateman AW. Drug treatment for personality disorders. Adv Psychiatr Treat 2004; 10:389–98

Further reading

Cloninger CR, Svrakic DM, Pryzbeck TR. A psychobiological model of temperament and character. Arch Gen Psychiatry 1993; 50: 975–90

Gillies D, Beck A, McCloud A, Rathbone J. Benzodiazepines alone or in combination with antipsychotic drugs for acute psychosis. Cochrane Database Syst Rev 2005; CD003079

Huf G, Alexander J, Allen MH. Haloperidol plus promethazine for psychosis induced aggression. Cochrane Database Syst Rev 2004; CD005146

McAllister-Williams RH, Ferrier IN. Rapid tranquillisation: time for a reappraisal of options for parenteral therapy. Br J Psychiatry 2002; 180:485–9

Thompson C. The use of high-dose antipsychotic medication. Br J Psychiatry. 1994;164: 448–58 (Royal College of Psychiatrists consensus statement)

Zanarini MC, Frankenburg FR, Hennen J, Silk KR. The longitudinal course of borderline psychopathology: 6-year prospective follow-up of the phenomenology of borderline personality disorder. Am J Psychiatry 2003; 160:274–83

Drug treatment for childhood and adolescent disorders

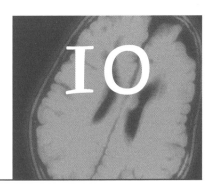

IO

David Coghill

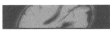 ## Background

■ Increased clinical interest in child and adolescent psychopharmacology has outstripped research, with the exception of attention deficit/hyperactivity disorder (ADHD).

■ This means that there is generally a lack of an evidence base on which to make prescribing decisions.

■ This is important, as children are not simply 'mini-adults':
  – their developing brains almost certainly react differently to psychoactive medication
  – differences in metabolism make it likely that they will display different side-effect profiles to those seen in adults.

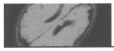 ## Attention deficit/hyperactivity disorder (ADHD)

Clinical background

■ The DSM-IV diagnosis of ADHD consists of:
  – extremes of *inattentive*, *impulsive* and *hyperactive* behaviour, which are
  – *pervasive*, of early *onset*, *unexplained* by other disorders, and result in *impairment* and *disability*.

■ ICD-10 'hyperkinetic disorder' is more restrictive, and requires more pervasive and impairing symptoms.

■ Epidemiology of ADHD:
  – the prevalence is 3–8% (hyperkinetic disorder around 1.5%)
  – it is three or four times more likely in boys than girls
  – it is highly comorbid: oppositional defiant disorder and conduct disorder are most common.

■ Only a small proportion of those with ADHD are identified, diagnosed and treated.

- ADHD is a chronic condition:
  - it commonly continues through adolescence and into adulthood
  - if untreated, it is associated with educational and employment difficulties, relationship problems, increased accidents, substance misuse, and delinquency.

Scientific background

Although the aetiology of ADHD is incompletely understood, increasing evidence supports a biological basis.

Genetic studies

- Heritability of ADHD is estimated as greater than 0.8.
- Molecular genetics:
  - replicated evidence implicates dopamine (DA) genes (D_4, D_5, the DA transporter)
  - preliminary evidence implicates D_1 and 5-HT_{1B}, dopamine-β-hydroxylase (DβH), and SNAP-25 (involved in the regulation of neurotransmitter release)
  - it is polygenic, with a small contribution from each gene (odds ratios 1.2–1.9).

Brain imaging and electrophysiology

- Structural/functional abnormalities have been shown in frontal, temporal and parietal cortical regions, basal ganglia, callosal areas, and cerebellum.
- Abnormalities are evident early in development, are nonprogressive and are not a consequence of stimulant treatment.

Neuropsychology

- Studies demonstrate deficits in higher-order cognitive functions, including working memory and inhibition, motivational processes, memory, timing, and time perception.

Neurotransmitters

There is converging evidence for catecholamine dysregulation from:

- animal models
- molecular genetic findings
- functional imaging studies
- the effectiveness of stimulants (related to DA) and noradrenaline (NA) drugs in treatment.

Management of ADHD

- Multimodal intervention is usually indicated, and should target both the core ADHD symptoms and associated or comorbid problems.
- Psychological and educational interventions, medication, and diet should all be available, and their use should be guided by an individualised treatment plan.

Non-pharmacological treatments

- Psychoeducational measures:
  - education and advice should be the basis of any treatment offered.
- Parent training and behavioural interventions in the family:
  - effectiveness has been shown in randomised controlled trials (RCTs)
  - there are many approaches, and evidence-based treatment manuals are available.
- Behavioural interventions (preschool or school):
  - these are effective in reducing hyperactive behaviour and promoting social adjustment
  - no one scheme has been shown to be superior to others.

Pharmacological treatments

Stimulant drugs

These have been used to treat ADHD symptoms since 1937.

Methylphenidate and dexamfetamine

- Mechanism of action (see also Chapter 1):
  - methylphenidate is a DA transporter blocker
  - dexamfetamine blocks the DA transporter and stimulates synaptic DA release
  - both drugs increase DA levels in the nucleus accumbens and therefore have abuse potential (see Chapter 7). However, the best available evidence suggests that treatment of ADHD with stimulants reduces rather than increases the likelihood of later substance misuse.
- The pharmacokinetic, pharmacodynamic and clinical effects of both drugs are very similar:
  - they have a short half-life ($t_{1/2}$ = 3 hours), rapid onset of action (t_{max} = 1.5 hours) and short duration of action (3–4 hours)
  - immediate-release forms require multiple daily dosing (two or three times per day)

- extended-release preparations are becoming available with increased duration of action (8–12 hours, depending on the preparation). As of early 2006, two extended-release methylphenidate preparations are available in the UK. One (Concerta XL) uses an osmotic pump system (OROS) to deliver methylphenidate over a 12-hour period, while the other (Equasym XL) uses time-release beads to deliver methylphenidate over an 8-hour period.
- Efficacy:
  - short-term efficacy and effectiveness at reducing core ADHD symptoms has been established in a large number of clinical trials and meta-analyses (mean effect size 0.9). They are effective in around 70% of cases, with around 95% having a clinically meaningful response to one drug or the other
  - they are rapidly effective: a response is seen after the first dose
  - evidence for longer-term efficacy is much weaker, as there are no truly long-term trials of stimulant treatment of ADHD.
- Side-effects:
  - most common are decreased appetite and insomnia (dose-related)
  - less common are depression, irritability, increase in tics and raised blood pressure
  - rare side-effects are rash, allergic reactions, blood dyscrasias, hepatotoxicity, and possibly serious cardiovascular events.
- Monitoring of height, weight pulse and blood pressure is recommended.
- Drug interactions: see Table 10.1.
- Prescribing issues
  - despite continuing public and media controversy, there is little evidence that methylphenidate or dexamfetamine are associated with any negative long-term treatment outcomes in ADHD
  - large interindividual variation requires wide dose titration to achieve a balance between symptom reduction and side-effects
  - the requirement to take medication three times a day, and during school, can lead to practical and compliance problems, stigma, and restriction in activities. Extended-release stimulant preparations may reduce some of these problems
  - the decision as to whether medication should be started will depend on the presentation of each individual case (Table 10.2).
- Guidance
  - in the UK, the Scottish Intercollegiate Guidelines Network (SIGN) and the National Institute for Clinical Excellence (NICE) regard methylphenidate and dexamfetamine as first-line treatments of ADHD. This is subject to diagnosis, initiation and management being carried out by specialists in ADHD within a shared care protocol with primary care, with at least 6-monthly monitoring

Table 10.1 Selected drug interactions with stimulant drugs

Action/effect	Drug/drug class
Inhibition of metabolism/increased plasma concentration of named drug	TCAs
	SSRIs
	Some anticonvulsants (phenobarbital, phenytoin, primidone)
Decreased therapeutic effect of named drugs	Antipsychotics
	Adrenergic neuron blockers (antihypertensive action)
Hypertension	MAOIs
	Oxytocin
	Doxapram
Increased plasma concentration of methylphenidate	Some anticonvulsants (phenobarbital, phenytoin, primidone)
Sudden death (?: causal link not established)	Clonidine

TCA, tricyclic antidepressant; SSRI, selective serotonin reuptake inhibitor; MAOI, monoamine oxidase inhibitor.

Table 10.2 Factors to consider before prescribing medication for attention deficit/hyperactivity disorder (ADHD)

- A diagnosis of ADHD or hyperkinetic disorder is required
- Are symptoms pervasive across all situations?
  - If not, psychosocial interventions specific to situation should be given as the first treatment option. Consider stimulants after a reasonable failed trial (e.g. 3 months)
  - In those with severe pervasive ADHD/hyperkinetic disorder, medication can be considered as first choice treatment with or without psychosocial interventions, depending on individual circumstances
  - If medication is to be used, a short-acting stimulant will usually be the first choice; however, there are situations where it is appropriate to initiate treatment with an extended-release stimulant or atomoxetine
- Age:
  - Preschool children: methylphenidate is not licensed below 6 years; evidence for efficacy of stimulants is less secure
  - Adolescents: possible lower response rates, problems with compliance and increased risk of drug misuse
  - Adults: less evidence for efficacy of stimulants, lower response rate and increased risk of drug misuse. Nonstimulants may be considered earlier in the treatment pathway
- Attitudes of patient and carers to drug treatment

- the influential Multimodal Treatment Study of ADHD (the MTA study) demonstrated the superiority of a carefully managed and structured medication package over both behavioural treatment and unstructured community-based pharmacological treatment. Components included more intensive medication regime, blind initial dose titration, supportive counselling and reading materials, and monthly consultations for dose adjustment.

Pemoline

- This is a longer-acting stimulant with main actions due to inhibition of DA reuptake.
- It has comparable effectiveness to methylphenidate and dexamfetamine.
- The UK and US licences for ADHD have been withdrawn due to severe liver toxicity in a number of patients.

Adderall and Adderall XR

- These are extended-release mixed amfetamine salt preparations containing 25% levoamfetamine and 75% dextroamfetamine.
- Efficacy has been demonstrated for the treatment of ADHD symptoms in several RCTs.
- Adderall is an immediate-release preparation that may have a small but statistically significant efficacy advantage over immediate-release methylphenidate. Adderall appears to have a longer duration of action than immediate-release methylphenidate from comparative studies.
- Adderall XR is an extended-release preparation based on bead technology and designed to be effective over a 12-hour period.
- Both preparations are licensed for the treatment of ADHD in the USA, but not in the UK.

Non-stimulant drugs

Only atomoxetine is licensed for use in ADHD in the UK. Modafanil has recently received a license for use in the treatment of ADHD in the USA.

Atomoxetine

- This is a highly specific NA reuptake inhibitor.
- It affects DA as well as NA function, and it is likely that clinical effects are associated with both effects.
- There is no alteration of DA levels in the nucleus accumbens; thus atomoxetine is unlikely to be associated with abuse potential.
- It is metabolised by hepatic cytochrome P450 2D6, but no association between poor-metaboliser status and increased adverse events has been reported.

- All published industry-sponsored placebo-controlled RCTs in ADHD in children, adolescents and adults have reported that atomoxetine is superior to placebo in reduction of core ADHD symptoms (mean effect size 0.7).
- Currently available data directly comparing atomoxetine and stimulant medications are difficult to interpret due to the design of the studies. However, stimulants appear to have a greater effect size than atomoxetine.
- Although the plasma $t_{1/2}$ of atomoxetine is short (approximately 4 hours), the behavioural effects last longer than predicted from the pharmacokinetics, and once-daily dosing is effective, with the effects lasting across the whole day.
- Effects may be seen early, but take 8–12 weeks to maximise.
- Adverse effects:
  - the main ones are decreased appetite, vomiting, nausea, dizziness, asthenia and dyspepsia
  - hepatotoxicity, an increased risk of seizures and QTc prolongation has recently been identified
  - an analysis of 12 short-term studies found an increased risk of suicidal thinking compared with placebo among children with ADHD, but not adults.
- Atomoxetine is generally considered after either non-response to or failure to tolerate stimulant treatment; however, it may be considered as first-line treatment where substance misuse is a problem, where there is a particular need to control symptoms in the late evening or early morning, or where there is a particular patient/parent desire to avoid stimulant medication.

Modafanil

- This is a structurally and pharmacologically unique wake-promoting agent available in the UK for improving wakefulness in patients with excessive sleepiness associated with narcolepsy, obstructive sleep apnea and shiftwork sleep disorder.
- It promotes wakefulness that is distinct from amfetamines.
- Action on brain sites involved in 'normal' wakefulness:
  - hypothalamic mechanism
  - minimal generalised central nervous system (CNS) excitation.
- Enhancement of hypothalamocortical pathways results in maintenance of activity in the cortex, including the prefrontal cortex, which in turn leads to activation of neurons involved in higher-order functions such as reasoning, abstraction, planning and initiating activity, shaping of behavior patterns, prioritizing actions, and coordinating motor and sensory functions into a goal-directed stream of behaviours.
- It has demonstrated efficacy in treating ADHD in three industry-sponsored studies (mean effect size 0.7).
- The main side-effects are insomnia, headache, appetite decrease and abdominal pain.
- It has low abuse potential.

■   There have been rare reports of serious skin reactions (including suspected cases of both erythema multiforme and Stevens–Johnson syndrome).

Tricyclic antidepressants (TCAs)

■   These were previously recommended in the UK as third-line treatment for ADHD, but have been used less frequently since the introduction of atomoxetine.
■   TCAs are associated with a wide range of side-effects and are toxic in overdose (see Chapter 4), and should be used with extreme caution in children and adolescents.
■   In terms of efficacy, a systematic review concluded that:
    –   studies comparing stimulants with TCAs had many limitations
    –   desipramine is more effective than placebo (but has been withdrawn from the market in the UK due to concerns over cardiotoxicity)
    –   imipramine shows inconsistent results, and there are at present insufficient data on which to base judgements.

Other nonstimulant preparations

The following have been used in treating ADHD, but there are insuffient data to assess efficacy:

■   clonidine
■   bupropion
■   guanfacine
■   venlafaxine (contraindicated in children and adolescents).

 # Autism

Background

■   Autism is a pervasive developmental disorder consisting of qualitative impairment of social functioning and communication, and restricted, repetitive and stereotyped patterns of behaviour and interests.
■   The understanding of its complex aetiology remains incomplete, but there is evidence for reduced 5-HT neurotransmission and altered DA neurotransmission.
■   Educational and behavioural treatments remain the mainstay of therapy for children and adolescents with autism.

Drug treatments for autism

There is increased interest in the role of medication as an adjunctive therapy for specific troublesome behaviours (rather than core symptoms), namely hyperactivity, aggression, withdrawal, and repetitive, ritualised, stereotyped or self-injurious behaviours.

Antidepressants

Drugs primarily affecting 5-HT neurotransmission may show efficacy:

▪ Clomipramine has been demonstrated to be superior to placebo and desipramine on ratings of autistic symptoms (including stereotypies), anger, and compulsive, ritualised behaviours.
▪ Adverse events associated with clomipramine, including QTc prolongation, tachycardia and seizures, mean that it must be used with great care in this population.
▪ Fluvoxamine was superior to placebo in one study in reducing repetitive thoughts and behaviour, maladaptive behaviour, and aggression. It also improved some aspects of social relatedness, particularly language use. However, another RCT has reported no difference between fluvoxamine and placebo.

Antipsychotics

Critics of the use of antipsychotics in children with autism suggest that they are being used merely as 'chemical straitjackets', but this does not seem to be the case.

Typical antipsychotics (DA antagonists)

▪ Haloperidol has been the most intensely studied psychopharmacologic agent for children and adolescents with autism.
▪ Several RCTs have demonstrated haloperidol to be effective in reducing a wide range of maladaptive behaviours in children and adolescents with autism, including hyperactivity, withdrawal, aggression and temper tantrums, stereo-typies and mood lability. It has also been demonstrated to increase social relatedness and discriminant learning.
▪ These positive effects need to be balanced against the frequent and disabling adverse reactions:
  – in the short term, excessive sedation and extrapyramidal side-effects are common
  – approximately one-third of children suffer from withdrawal dyskinesias and around 10% may develop tardive dyskinesia.
▪ As a result, despite its proven effectiveness, many clinicians remain wary about using haloperidol in autism.

Atypical antipsychotics (combined DA and 5-HT antagonists)

▪ Clinical trial data support the use of risperidone, olanzapine and quetiapine in the treatment of autism.

- They seem to be effective and well tolerated for the treatment of tantrums, aggression and self-injurious behaviour.
- Increased appetite and weight gain, fatigue, drowsiness, dizziness, and drooling are common with risperidone.
- Relatively small doses appear effective and seem independent of common adverse events such as drowsiness and fatigue.

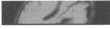 # Depressive disorders

- Psychotherapeutic interventions, particularly cognitive–behavioural therapy (CBT) and interpersonal therapy (IPT) are effective in the treatment of many children and adolescents with depressive symptoms and mild to moderate depressive episodes and should probably be considered first-line treatment.
- Psychopharmacological interventions for juvenile depression have been the subject of extreme scrutiny over the past 2 years, with concerns being raised questioning both their safety and their efficacy. Medication is, however, indicated for moderate to severe depressive disorders where effective psychosocial interventions are impractical or where depression fails to respond to an adequate trial of psychotherapy of at least 3 months. Drug treatments should not be used as the sole intervention, and should be only initiated after consultation with a child and adolescent psychiatrist.
- See Chapter 4 for details of antidepressants.

Tricyclic antidepressants (TCAs)

- TCAs are of unlikely benefit in the treatment of depression in prepubertal children.
- There is marginal evidence to support the use of TCAs in the treatment of depression in adolescents, but benefits are likely to be moderate at best.
- Side-effects and toxicity in overdose mean that extreme caution is required in their use.

Selective serotonin reuptake inhibitors (SSRIs) and selective noradrenaline reuptake inhibitors (SNRIs)

- There has been a rapid increase in the use of SSRIs in children and adolescents, which has outstripped the evidence base.
- While these newer antidepressants have been used to treat childhood and adolescent depression, RCTs have not demonstrated unequivocal benefits of antidepressant medication over placebo.
- A systematic review that examined the risk–benefit profile of SSRIs and SNRIs in the treatment of childhood depression concluded that fluoxetine has

demonstrated a favourable risk–benefit profile, whereas for the other SSRIs and SNRIs the risks outweigh benefits.

- Major concerns regarding adverse effects of antidepressants – particularly suicidal thought and hostility – have led both the UK and US regulatory authorities to issue warnings about the use of these medications in patients under 18 years of age.
- The NICE guideline for the assessment and treatment of depression in children and young people (2005) recommends:
  - psychological intervention should be the first-line treatment
  - medication should only be considered in cases of moderate or severe depression unresponsive to psychological intervention
  - fluoxetine should be the first-line pharmacological treatment
  - where fluoxetine is not tolerated or is unsuccessful, sertraline or citalopram should be the second-line pharmacological treatment
  - in psychotic depression, consideration should be given to augmenting antidepressant treatment with an atypical antipsychotic.
- None of these drugs currently have UK Marketing Authorisation for use in depression in children and adolescents under the age of 18 years.

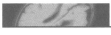 ## Manic episodes and bipolar disorder

- There is considerable confusion and disagreement over the most appropriate ways in which to diagnose manic episodes and bipolar disorder in child and adolescent populations.
- In the UK, a diagnosis of bipolar disorder is still rarely made (it is much more common in the USA).
- It is very difficult to know exactly which patients have been included in clinical trials for the treatment of early-onset bipolar disorder and how to translate this into clinical practice.
- Nevertheless, it does seem to be the case that true manic episodes are difficult to treat without medication.
- There is some evidence from case series and open-label trials for the efficacy of lithium, valproate/valproate semisodium and carbamazepine in the treatment of early-onset mania.
- A small RCT showed that adding quetiapine to valproate is more effective than valproate alone for the treatment of mania in adolescents.

Obsessive–compulsive disorder (OCD)

- The SSRIs sertraline and fluvoxamine have both been demonstrated to be safe and effective treatments for paediatric OCD, and are licensed for use in children and adolescents in the UK.
- Long-term treatment is well tolerated and effective at maintaining improvement, with continued improvement for up to 1 year.

- Obsessional symptoms may relapse on discontinuation of treatment, but it is suggested that withdrawal of treatment should be attempted after 1–1.5 years and restarted if significant symptoms reoccur.
- Paediatric OCD may not respond as well to some SSRIs as does adult OCD:
  - 20–25% are symptom-free at the end of a course of treatment, 20–50% have some improvement and about 25% show no improvement.

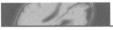

Anxiety disorders

- The use of drug treatments in the management of child and adolescent anxiety disorders remains contentious, with many clinicians arguing that these disorders are most appropriately treated with psychosocial interventions.
- However, success rates for CBT are 70–80%, so significant numbers of children require further intervention.

Benzodiazepines

These are generally efficacious; however, adverse events and the risk of tolerance mean that they should only be considered when other pharmacological approaches have failed, and should only be prescribed for very short periods of time.

Tricyclic antidepressants (TCAs)

RCTs of TCAs conducted in paediatric anxiety have not demonstrated clear efficacy, and they should not be considered as first-line treatments for these disorders.

Selective serotonin reuptake inhibitors (SSRIs)

- Both fluvoxamine and sertraline have been reported in short-term RCTs to be efficacious in paediatric generalised anxiety disorder.
- Neither drug is licensed in this age group for this indication. In view of the recent decision to exclude their use in paediatric major depressive disorder, but to continue their use in paediatric OCD, it is not clear what the current status of guidance is for their prescription in anxiety disorders.

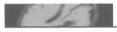

Guidelines

National Institute for Health and Clinical Excellence Technology Appraisal 98. Methylphenidate, atomoxetine and dexamfetamine for attention deficit hyperactivity disorder (ADHD) in children and adolescents (review), 2006. http://www.nice.org.uk/page.aspx?o=appraisals.completed

National Institute for Health and Clinical Excellence. Clinical Guideline 28. Depression in children and young people: identification and management in primary, community and secondary care, 2005. http://www.nice.org.uk/page.aspx?o=guidelines.completed

Scottish Intercollegiate Guidelines Network National Guideline 52. Attention deficit and hyperactivity disorders in children and young people, 2001. http://www.sign.ac.uk/guidelines/published/index.html

Taylor E, Döpfner M, Sergeant J et al. European clinical guidelines for hyperkinetic disorder – first upgrade. *Eur Child Adolesc Psychiatry* 2004; 13(Suppl 1):17–30

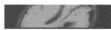 # References

Key references

Hazell P, O'Connell D, Heathcote D, Henry D. Tricyclic drugs for depression in children and adolescents. (Cochrane Review). In: The Cochrane Library, Issue 1, 2004

James AC, Javaloyes AM. The treatment of bipolar disorder in children and adolescents. J Child Psychol Psychiatry All Disciplines 2001; 42:439–49

Jureidini JN, Doecke CJ, Mansfield PR et al. Efficacy and safety of antidepressants for children and adolescents. BMJ 2004, 328:879–83

McCracken JT, McGough J, Shah B et al. Risperidone in children with autism and serious behavioral problems. N Engl J Med 2002, 347:314–21

MTA Co-operative Group. A 14-month randomized clinical trial of treatment strategies for attention-deficit/hyperactivity disorder. The MTA Co-operative Group. Multimodal Treatment Study of Children with ADHD. Arch Gen Psychiatry 1999, 56:1073–86

Riddle MA, Reeve EA, Yaryura-Tobias JA et al. Fluvoxamine for children and adolescents with obsessive-compulsive disorder: a randomized, controlled, multicenter trial. J Am Acad Child Adolesc Psychiatry 2001; 40:222–9

Whittington, C. J., Kendall, T., Fonagy, P et al. Selective serotonin reuptake inhibitors in child-hood depression: systematic review of published versus unpublished data. Lancet 2004, 363:1341–5

Further reading

British Association for Psychopharmacology. Child and learning disability psychopharma-cology. J Psychopharmacol 1997; 11:291–4

Eur Child Adolesc Psychiatry 2000; 9(Suppl 1) (This complete supplement comprises a series of excellent reviews on child and adolescent psychopharmacology)

Greenhill LL, Pliszka S, Dulcan MK et al, for the American Academy of Child and Adolescent Psychiatry. Practice parameter for the use of stimulant medications in the treatment of children, adolescents, and adults. J Am Acad Child Adolesc Psychiatry 2002, 41 (Suppl):26S-49S

MTA Co-operative Group. Moderators and mediators of treatment response for children with attention-deficit/hyperactivity disorder. The Multimodal Treatment Study of Children with ADHD. Arch Gen Psychiatry 1999; 56:1088–96

Psychopharmacology. Child Adolesc Psychiatric Clin North Am 2000; 9(1). (An entire volume devoted to the North American perspective on child and adolescent psychopharmacology)

Solanto MV, Arnsten AF, Castellanos FX. Stimulant Drugs and ADHD: Basic and Clinical Neuroscience. New York: Oxford University Press, 2001

Volkow ND, Swanson JM. Variables that affect the clinical use and abuse of methylphenidate in the treatment of ADHD. Am J Psychiatry 2003; 160:1909–18

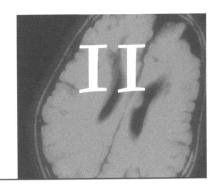

Clinical trial methodology

R Hamish McAllister-Williams and Stephen M Lawrie

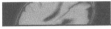 ## Introduction

- A general definition of 'clinical trial' is any kind of study designed to establish the effects of a particular therapeutic intervention.
- Table 11.1 gives some definitions of types of trials.

 ## History

- Clinical trials of some sort are probably as old as civilisation.
- James Lind, an 18th-century Scottish physician, is generally credited with having completed the first controlled trial – of vitamin C for scurvy.
- Early Nobel prizes in the field of psychiatry (Wagner-Jauregg in 1927 for 'malaria therapy' and Moniz in 1949 for the prefrontal leucotomy) were awarded for work that turned out to be ineffective and abused respectively.
- The gold standard of medical experimentation, the randomised control trial (RCT), was first used to evaluate the effects of antituberculous drugs in a trial sponsored by the UK Medical Research Council and published in 1948.
- There is increasing interest in designing valid naturalistic or pragmatic trials to determine effectiveness in usual clinical practice.

 ## Drug development

- New drugs can be developed:
  - by isolating the active ingredients in natural compounds
  - by modifying the chemistry of other drugs
  - from theoretical extension of basic scientific knowledge.
- Only about 1 in every 10 000 potential products reach the market, often taking 10 years or more and many millions of pounds. Given the limited patent life (20 years in UK from the time of compound synthesis), drug companies often

Table 11.1 Some commonly used terms to describe types of trials

Term	Meaning
Controlled	A group receiving the investigative treatment is compared with another group receiving different treatment (e.g. placebo, no treatment or waiting list, another treatment of known efficacy). Usually applied to *prospective* (i.e. both groups are studied in parallel) rather than *retrospective* (i.e. using an historical control group treated at a previous time) trials
Placebo-controlled	One of the 'arms' of the trial is against a placebo condition. Usually required for a drug to be licensed
Randomised	Allocation to the different treatment 'arms' in the study is done randomly to minimise bias due to selection of patients for particular treatments
Open	Both clinician and patient know that a treatment is being given for a given indication. Open studies are usually uncontrolled (Note that in clinical practice this is often equivalent to giving a therapeutic trial for an unlicensed indication)
Single-blinded	Usually taken to indicate that the assessing clinicians, but not the patients, are informed about which treatment is being given[a]
Double-blinded	Neither the patient nor the assessing clinician are informed of which treatment is being given[a]
Triple-blinded	Used when there are separate treating clinicians and assessors, both of whom are blind to treatment allocation[a]
Naturalistic/pragmatic	Trials carried out in usual clinical practice, with trade-off between rigorous trial methodology and 'real-world' applicability
Non-inferiority	Trials statistically powered to be able to detect a prespecified difference between two active drugs that is judged to be clinically significant

[a] It is usually not checked/made clear whether blinding is successful in practice.

adopt aggressive marketing strategies to recoup their costs and deliver profits for shareholders.

- A new drug is first tested in animals, to establish the potential for desired effects and absence of unexpected or undesirable effects, before going through the four phases in humans (Table 11.2).
- Phase I trials determine basic pharmacological parameters in human volunteers (e.g. pharmacokinetics, adverse effects, tolerance):
  - they are usually open or uncontrolled

Table 11.2   Phases of drug development

Phase	Question addressed	Main methods
Preclinical	Pharmacology and toxicology	Biochemical and animal studies
I	Basic human pharmacology	Open/uncontrolled trials
II	Efficacy in disease(s)	Controlled trials/small randomised controlled trials
III	Efficacy and comparative efficacy (for regulatory approval)	Randomised controlled trials
IV	Problems in clinical practice/ comparison with other drugs	Observational studies/randomised controlled trials

- adverse effects are often measured both subjectively and objectively (e.g. heart rate, blood pressure, neuropsychological, EEG)
- they generally require 24-hour clinical observations, and often exclude the young, women and the aged because effects in humans are unknown; however, a drug safe in adult men, for example, may not be safe in children, women and the aged
- because the studies are uncontrolled, some of the effects will be placebo effects.
- Phase II trials establish whether or not a given drug works in a variety of conditions:
  - they are usually controlled, in that some patients get placebo
  - in 'dose-ranging studies', to determine optimal dosage, each group of patients getting a particular dose of the drug can be thought of as a control group for the others.
- Phase III trials, sometimes called 'comparative' trials, seek to determine the effects of a new drug with reference to those commonly used in clinical practice:
  - they are usually randomised, with a proportion being placebo-controlled (a variety of other types of trial may be randomised and/or controlled, but these are rarely used in drug development studies – see below)
  - they tend to be larger than phase II studies
  - their major aim is to satisfy regulatory authorities and achieve a product licence.
- Phase IV clinical 'trials' refer to the various methods of surveillance (see below) to establish the frequency of any serious or unexpected adverse effects of a drug once it has been licensed and introduced into regular clinical practice:
  - they are similar to audit (measuring performance against a standard) and naturalistic outcome studies.

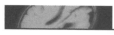 # Designing or appraising a clinical trial (Table 11.3)

What is the aim or hypothesis of the study?

Any study has a better chance of answering a single specific question rather than a number of less focused objectives. The question has to be:

- clinically relevant (i.e. the answer will help make therapeutic decisions)
- ethically acceptable (see below)
- not answered already (e.g. in a systematic review or meta-analysis), although replication of a finding in just one or two previous studies is reasonable.

Which patients are to be studied?

- This is a matter of stipulating criteria for inclusion and exclusion.
- Theoretically, there is tension between recruiting a 'pure' highly selected group and an unselected heterogeneous group. The former reduces variance in the data and hence can produce more reliable results, but the findings may not be representative of the entire patient population. The latter may be more valid, but it may be difficult to identify a given effect.
- In practice, broader inclusion criteria and minimal exclusions aid recruitment (particularly considering refusal and inability to give valid informed consent).
- Many psychiatric studies exclude patients with comorbid substance abuse – comprise about half of all the patients seen clinically:
  - this leaves uncertainty about efficacy in the comorbid group
  - it probably overestimates the benefits of any treatment in practice (noncompliance is high in comorbid patients).
- The usual practice of excluding patients younger than 16–18 and older than 60–65 years means that they often have to be treated without information from clinical trials, and usually 'off licence'.
- Involuntarily detained patients cannot be enrolled in clinical trials for ethical reasons, resulting in the most severely ill patients often being treated in the absence of reliable evidence.

Table 11.3 Questions relating to designing or appraising a clinical trial

1. What is the aim or hypothesis of the study?
2. Which patients are to be studied?
3. What intervention is being studied?
4. What type of clinical trial is appropriate?
5. Was randomisation appropriately carried out?
6. Which outcomes should be measured and how?
7. Were appropriate statistical tests used?

■ The trial setting determines the type of patients to whom the results will apply (inpatients, day patients, outpatients and/or those in primary care).

Which intervention is being studied?

■ Consider the type, formulation, dose, dosing schedule and route of administration of the medication.
■ Fixed versus flexible dosing:
  – results from fixed-dose trials are generally easier to interpret, but are different from how a drug is used in clinical practice, and many patients will receive non-optimal doses
  – results from flexible dosing (tailoring the dose to a particular patient) are more clinically representative, but can be difficult if the responsible clinician is blind to the treatment given.
■ What, if any, other drugs are permissible for participating patients – e.g. antipsychotic trials usually permit anticholinergic drugs and 'rescue' medication for behavioural disturbance.
■ Duration:
  – most trials are short (≤6 weeks), simply because they are easier to do (Fig. 11.1)
  – long trials are complex, expensive and liable to have large numbers of people dropping out. A dropout rate greater than 20% may mean dubious representativeness and reliability (but this is hard to avoid in many psychiatric studies, especially long-term ones)
  – ideally, clinical practice should be informed by long-term clinical trials, particularly if patients are advised to stay on a drug for 1 year or more – but this needs to be balanced against the likelihood of higher dropout rates.

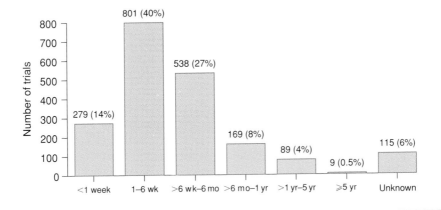

Figure 11.1 Duration of the first 2000 clinical trials in schizophrenia. (Reproduced by permission from Thornley B, Adams C. BMJ 1998; 317:1181–4.)

What type of clinical trial is appropriate?

Randomised controlled trials (RCTs) were devised to measure drug efficacy, and probably offer the greatest precision. However, they are not without problems, and alternative approaches may be sufficient or optimum, depending on the specific clinical question. RCTs measure clinical efficacy (how well a drug works under ideal conditions). Pragmatic (or naturalistic) trials measure clinical effectiveness (how well a drug works in usual clinical practice).

Nonspecific effects

Studies are inescapably confounded by nonspecific effects that lead to improvement in the absence of any specific pharmacological action of the drug being studied:

- Response rates on placebo can be very high (e.g. 30–40% in 8-week antidepressant studies).
- Placebo response rates in depression correlate positively with the year of study publication, i.e. rates are increasing. This is likely to apply to other disorders, and may relate to increasing use of more mildly ill patients (see below).
- These may lead to:
  - incorrect assumption of efficacy in uncontrolled trials
  - incorrect assumption of inefficacy in underpowered studies due to type II statistical errors
  - questioning of clinical significance even if statistical significance is attained, as a high response rate to placebo tends to lead to smaller drug-effect sizes.

There are three main components to the nonspecific response:

- Measurement effects:
  - whenever a population is chosen for an extreme characteristic above a specific cut-off (e.g. psychiatric rating score $> x$), a second measurement will tend to be less extreme simply because of less-than-perfect reliability in repeated measurement (called *regression to the mean*)
  - observer expectation: rating values may be elevated to include patients in a trial; subsequent ratings may be more objective or subject to expectation of improvement over time.
- Placebo effects (genuine but nonspecific treatment effects):
  - in RCTs, patients assigned to the placebo arm receive regular visits to their doctor and supportive help. This constitutes a treatment in its own right
  - patient (and doctor) expectations may engage a non-pharmacological healing process. This factor may be greater in more mildly ill patients and those with greater self-motivation recruited from advertisements.
- Spontaneous recovery is difficult to distinguish from a placebo effect and reflects the natural history of the disorder. It is likely to be greater in more mildly ill patients with shorter duration of illness.

Types of trials

- Uncontrolled trials:
  - these can establish whether a treatment works at all and the profile of adverse effects
  - however, nonspecific/placebo effects cannot be excluded in the absence of a control group.
- Controlled trials:
  - these allow evaluation against placebo or a pre-existing treatment
  - they may reduce or control for placebo effects
  - in the absence of randomisation, they are still subject to selection bias (conscious or unconscious). Patients getting a new treatment tend to be less severely ill and/or have better prognosis. Beneficial effects of new drugs are typically overestimated by 30–40%.
- RCTs:
  - randomisation increases the scientific quality or 'internal validity' of a trial (see below)
  - there are problems with 'external validity', i.e. patients able to give informed consent and willing to be randomized tend to differ from many potential participants. This limits their representativeness, and hence the generalisability of the results to all patients
  - RCTs designed to show a greater effect than placebo (with sufficient statistical power) are required to establish efficacy. RCTs against comparator drugs are frequently too poorly powered to be able to show a difference, and claims of equal efficacy need to be treated with caution. Recently, so-called *non-inferiority* studies have been used in this situation. These are designed to have sufficient statistical power to detect a predefined difference between drugs, which is believed to be of clinical importance (see 'Power calculation' below).
- Pragmatic trials:
  - these have more external but less internal validity
  - patient groups are representative, the interventions are routinely feasible and outcome measures are clinically relevant
  - one option is to enrol patients for whom the clinician is uncertain as to which treatment should be prescribed
  - pragmatic trials are increasingly being applied in psychiatry.
- Patient preference trials:
  - these are a specific type of pragmatic trial
  - patients not willing to be randomised are given their preferred treatment They are followed up as in the trial, and their results are compared with those who were randomised.
- Crossover trials:
  - all participants receive two (or more) interventions one after the other, with the two groups receiving a different treatment first
  - these are useful in relatively rare diseases where small numbers do not permit an RCT.

- however, it is difficult to ensure that the trial is long enough to see therapeutic effects but short enough to avoid natural fluctuations confounding the trial
- there is also the problem of carry-over effects from the first treatment period to the second, and the potential for drug interactions
- 'wash-out periods' of no treatment introduce new difficulties with sudden cessation of potentially effective treatments.

- *N*-of-1 trials:
  - these are crossover trials in which a patient is given two treatments. They may be useful if it is not known which treatment the patient may benefit from
  - they require patient consent and cooperation from the hospital pharmacy.

- Audit and naturalistic outcome studies:
  - these are not usually thought of as clinical trials, but are similar to phase IV 'trials'
  - they are uncontrolled, and are therefore unreliable even if patients are used as their own 'historical control'
  - nevertheless, they may provide valuable effectiveness information.

Was randomisation carried out appropriately?

- There are two main purposes of randomisation:
  - to evenly distribute known and unknown confounders (e.g. age, sex, prognostic factors) affecting outcome
  - to avoid selection bias (depends on concealing allocation).

- Successful randomisation is inversely related to the chance of a trial finding a treatment effect (in one review, 58% of randomized studies, where allocation could have been compromised, found a benefit of the new treatment, versus 9% of randomised trials with adequate allocation concealment).

- Note that allocation concealment in randomisation is different to blinding (Table 11.1).

- Allocation concealment:
  - requires an unpredictable randomisation schedule, i.e. not dates of birth, day of week, etc.
  - otherwise, investigators may consciously or unconsciously subvert randomisation.

- Ideally, randomisation consists of:
  - assignment by random numbers (tossing a coin is acceptable)
  - treatment assignment only being revealed after consent to participate has been obtained (preferably by an independent person)
  - methods including sealed opaque envelopes or telephoning a centralised allocation unit.

- Randomisation methods to ensure that trial groups are balanced in terms of number and/or patient characteristics:
  - patients are '*blocked*' in groups (of four, six, etc.) to ensure broadly equal numbers in groups

- they are *'stratified'* to ensure that possible prognostic factors (e.g. age, sex, duration of illness) are balanced – this requires a randomisation schedule for each stratum
- *'minimisation'* is applied, in which subsequent patients are allocated by minimising differences in important variables.
- Cluster trials are those in which subjects are randomised in groups or clusters – this is most common for wider aspects of health services than one particular treatment, e.g. effects of education on general practitioners done by group practice. The main disadvantage is that the unit of randomisation should be the unit of analysis, requiring large numbers of individuals for adequate power.

Which outcomes should be measured, and how?

- Clinical outcomes can be measured either categorically (e.g. recovered/not recovered) or continuously (e.g. symptom severity scales).
- Categorical outcomes:
  - are easiest to understand, and are potentially the most clinically meaningful
  - however, they may be determined from arbitrary cut-off points on rating scales or other measures (e.g. response measured as a percentage reduction in symptom severity). This can lead to spurious findings of apparently large effects as a result of clinically insignificant changes in overall symptoms (see the paper by Moncrieff and Kirsch (2005) and the response)
  - require nonparametric statistics.
- Outcomes:
  - these should be prespecified (typically symptom severity scores, but might include adverse effects, drop-outs, quality-of-life measures, etc.)
  - multiple outcome measures increase the likelihood of finding statistically significant differences by chance.
- Ratings scales:
  - if observer-rated scales are used, these should be reliable (when rated by two or more observers) and should be sensitive to change
  - psychiatry has had a surfeit of rating scales, making comparison between trials problematic
  - researchers who use self-devised scales are more likely to report statistically significant effects than if they use standard measures.
- Blinding:
  - the aim is to reduce bias and placebo effects (Table 11.1)
  - it is rarely entirely successful (response or side-effects may reveal which treatment has been given)
  - independent outcome assessors may mitigate these problems to some degree

- success of blinding can be checked by asking participants/assessors which treatment they believed they received. However, this can be complicated by subjects equating success with active treatment. If there is a large benefit to the active treatment, subjects may guess on the basis of outcome – not because the blind has been broken.

Were appropriate statistical tests used?

- ▦ Effect size and significance:
  - care should be taken to distinguish between statistical and clinical significance
  - clinical significance relates to the magnitude of the effect size (e.g. is the advantage of the drug over placebo great enough to be clinically relevant?)
  - because of the potential problem with categorical outcomes (see above), clinical significance may be better assessed from mean endpoint rating scale scores
  - the effect size needed to reach clinical significance is arbitrarily determined (e.g. for depression, NICE defined this to be 3 points on the Hamilton Depression Rating scale for first-line antidepressant treatment versus placebo)
  - the smaller the effect size, the larger the sample needed to have a chance of detecting a statistically significant effect (see 'Power calculation' below) Beware of large samples with statistically significant but clinically irrelevant findings. (Note that on its own, the size of the p-value is not an indicator of the effect size or clinical significance)
  - it has been argued that, because of large (and increasing) placebo response rates in RCTs and the highly selected patients who are entered, the only meaningful way of assessing the clinical effect size of an intervention is through large pragmatic studies. RCTs may only indicate whether two treatments are statistically different, rather than the clinical importance.
- ▦ Power calculation:
  - this is necessary to determine the number of participants needed to detect a given finding at a specified level of statistical significance. This requires a defined primary outcome measure with estimation of numbers achieving a categorical outcome or likely mean difference continuous measure with its likely variance
  - it is standard to aim for 90% power to detect a given effect size with $p < 0.05$ difference, but different values can be specified. Various methods are available to calculate this (e.g. tables, computerised statistical packages).
- ▦ Size of trial:
  - most early RCTs in depression or schizophrenia had fewer than 60 participants (Fig. 11.2). This is just about adequate to identify significant

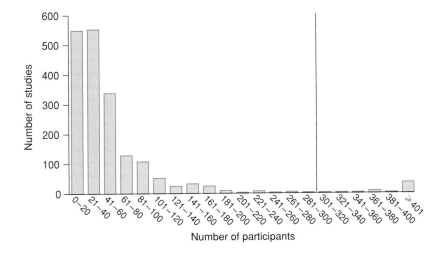

Figure 11.2   The size of the first 2000 controlled trials in schizophrenia. The line indicates the number of patients required to find a 20% difference between treatments with standard power. (Reproduced by permission from Thornley B, Adams C. BMJ 1998; 317:1181–4.)

        differences between an active treatment and placebo, depending on the effect size
- trials comparing two active agents require much larger groups, as the difference is generally much smaller
- larger trials more accurately measure outcomes, because the patients are likely to be more representative, measurement error is reduced, and they tend to be better planned and organised
- very large (mega) trials, including thousands of patients, are the best way of asking important therapeutic questions, but there is a risk that small, clinically insignificant, differences will be found.

Types of analysis:
- the particular statistical tests used depend on the properties of the data
- continuous measures provide more statistical power than categorical ones. The latter have advantages when dealing with dropouts from the trial before completion
- in intention-to-treat (ITT) analysis, all randomised participants are included, i.e. including treatment dropouts. With categorical measures, dropouts are usually assigned to the poor-outcome group. This may under- or overestimate efficacy, and is difficult to interpret if there is a high dropout rate or if the rate differs between treatments
- last observation carried forward (LOCF) analysis is the standard approach with a continuous measure, using the last available measure as the final measure. This may be ITT if it includes baseline data or may only include subjects who have completed a certain period of treatment (e.g. 2 weeks). It may over- or underestimate efficacy (Fig. 11.3)

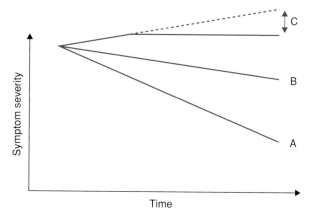

Figure 11.3 The responses of three hypothetical participants in a trial. Patient A has a good response and B a minimal improvement, and C drops out as the condition is deteriorating. In this case, in a last observation carried forward (LCOF) analysis, overall symptom deterioration will be underestimated by the size of the arrow and the treatment will appear better – especially with large numbers of dropouts. However, depending on the disorder, the opposite is possible; if dropouts are due to improvement or incidental factors then these patients may also improve, and sometimes the numbers deteriorating and improving after dropout will be equal. The point here is that it is simply not known what has happened to these people.

- it has recently been suggested that a likelihood-based mixed effects model repeated measures (MMRM) approach gives a better estimate of outcome than the traditional LOCF approach. This models the time-course for missing data rather than carrying forward the last value unchanged. It may be more robust than LOCF and avoid both under- and overestimates of treatment effect with the latter
- completer analysis includes only those who are still in the trial at the end. This overestimates treatment effects and is generally to be avoided.
- Problematic analyses:
  - the success of randomisation should not be tested by comparing descriptive variables: some will differ by chance
  - subgroups of patients can be defined by who responded particularly well or badly to treatment and taking this to indicate that certain groups should get particular treatments. The exception is if there was a prespecified hypothesis. Subgroup analysis is acceptable if it is clearly presented as exploratory, i.e. for future hypothesis testing
  - multiple hypothesis testing: one statistical comparison in 20 is likely to be significant at $p < 0.05$ by chance alone. This is acceptable if there are prespecified hypotheses, but correction for multiple testing should be made. Exploratory testing ('data dredging') is acceptable if it is clearly stated as such

- Meta-analysis:
  - individual RCTs and pragmatic primary research studies are prone to bias, random variation and type II errors. Meta-analysis is a method of pooling results from individual studies to increase power
  - they must be part of a systematic review to attempt to get all relevant studies to avoid selection bias; nevertheless, publication bias is possible, as negative RCTs may be unpublished
  - the methods of study selection, data extraction and subsequent combination can vary tremendously and can greatly influence the conclusions that are drawn
  - evidence-based medicine projects such as the Cochrane Collaboration aim to improve the registration of clinical trials and the synthesis of results (http://www.cochrane.org).

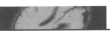 # Ethical considerations

- Ethical issues apply to all stages of any trial – the Declaration of Helsinki (Fifth Revision) applies.
- Planning a trial:
  - the trial should address an unresolved question
  - the methods employed should be likely to provide a useful answer (e.g. be sufficiently powered)
  - a recent issue has been the ethics of placebo control in conditions such as schizophrenia and depression where standard treatments are effective
  - attention needs to be paid to what treatment is offered at the termination of the trial, particularly if patients have been treated with placebo
  - ethical approval is required, with patient information and consent forming an important aspect of the application
  - drugs unlicensed for a particular indication need specific trial approval from the regulatory authorities (the Medicines and Healthcare Products Regulatory Authority in the UK), with regulations implementing the European Union Directive on Good Clinical Practice in Clinical Trials (2001).
- Consent:
  - fully informed, usually written, consent is required: participants should fully appreciate the nature of the trial and the potential risks and benefits
  - this may be a particular problem in psychiatry, with recent concerns about consent even in relatively stable psychotic patients: this appears to be related to cognitive impairment and can be dealt with by appropriate education
  - third-party consent may be appropriate good practice if a participant cannot consent, but this lacks legal force and is likely to reduce enrolment.
- Conduct of trial:
  - good clinical practice guidelines apply: e.g Association of British Pharmaceutical Industry Guidelines and EU Directives

- payments or inducements are not allowed, but compensation can be given (e.g. for travel and subsistence). Healthy volunteers can also receive compensation for inconvenience or discomfort
- insurance or indemnity agreement may be necessary for adverse effects
- research data are confidential, and should be stored anonymously and safely.

▓ Fraudulent analysis or presentation of results of a trial is unethical, and may be misleading or dangerous.

▓ In the UK, there has been a reform of Ethics Committees, which in 2004 became legally accountable to the UK Ethics Committee Authority with a unified application system. There is debate about the balance to be struck between protecting research subjects and increased restrictions and bureaucracy discouraging research.

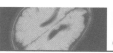 Postmarketing surveillance/phase IV clinical trials

Some important adverse effects detected by postmarketing surveillance are shown in Table 11.4.

Table 11.4 Some important adverse effects detected by post-marketing surveillance

Year	Drug	Adverse effect
1961	Thalidomide	Phocomelia[a]
1963	MAOIs	Cheese reactions
1976	Clozapine	Agranulocytosis[b]
1979–90	Mianserin	Blood dyscrasia[b]
1983	Zimelidine	Hypersensitivity reactions and Guillain–Barré syndrome[a]
1986	Nomifensine	Haemolytic anaemia[a]
1990	Pimozide	Ventricular arrythmias[b]
1993	Remoxipride	Aplastic anaemia[a]
1998	Sertindole	Possibility of sudden (cardiac) death[a]
1999	Vigabatrin	Visual field defects[b]
2001	Droperidol	QT prolongation on ECG[a]
2001	Thioridazine	QT prolongation on ECG[a]
2003	Nefazodone	Hepatotoxicity[a] ([b] in USA)

[a] Leading to product withdrawal (or highly restricted use).
[b] Leading to requirements for appropriate monitoring (and usually restricted use as well).

Voluntary reporting

- This depends upon the observational skills and conscientiousness of individual clinicians.
- Countries have national reporting systems. In the UK, the Committee for the Safety of Medicines/Medicine and Healthcare Products Regulatory Agency (http://www.mhra.gov.uk) encourages notification of possible adverse reactions, especially for new products (indicated by 'black triangles'), using the 'Yellow Card Scheme'. This was extended in 2005 to patients, who can report adverse events using the Patient Yellow Card Scheme (http://www.yellow card.gov.uk).
- National centres can send such information to the World Health Organisation (WHO) Collaborating Centre for International Drug Monitoring.
- The method:
  - is cheap
  - probably underestimates serious adverse effects and is inadequate as an epidemiological tool
  - has identified adverse effects resulting in withdrawal of particular products (e.g. remoxipride).

Intensive surveillance

- More intensive surveillance is expensive and usually restricted to hospital inpatients.
- Examples include the Boston Collaborative Drug Surveillance Programme (http://www.bu.edu/bcdsp) and the Medicines Evaluation and Monitoring Group (MEMO) in the UK.

Retrospective studies

- These are more expensive, but are much more informative than simple voluntary systems.
- Drawbacks are selection bias and unavailability of information.
- Examples include:
  - simple case–control studies
  - the Retrospective Assessment of Drug Safety (RADS) programme
  - pre-existing data storage systems, such as Office of Population Censuses and Surveys (OPCS) data
  - the recent report by the UK-based General Practice Research Database of an increased risk of venous thromboembolism on antipsychotic drugs.
- Databases can be linked by computer (e.g. people exposed to a particular product and people admitted to hospital with a particular problem). Linking a national registry of clozapine recipients to national death records found that clozapine increased the risk of fatal pulmonary embolism and respiratory disorders, but reduced the risk of suicide.

Prospective studies

- These are the most reliable – but also the most expensive.
- Examples:
  - a new product may be released with recorded/registered prescriptions to facilitate monitoring
  - an established product can be monitored (e.g. prompted blood tests with clozapine)
  - prescription event monitoring (PEM): a standard cohort study of the first 10 000 patients exposed to a particular drug. This is sufficiently powerful to detect an adverse reaction risk of 0.1%, but relies on accurate reporting and has been known to miss important adverse effects.

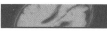 Conclusions

- Patients need protection from unscrupulous or overenthusiastic triallists, but trials are needed to establish effective new treatments.
- The 'explanatory' RCT has given clinical therapeutics a sound scientific base, but measures efficacy rather than effectiveness.
- Pragmatic clinical trials and multicentre studies in psychiatry are in their infancy, but have much to commend them in determining effectiveness in clinical practice.
- Single trials can be cited to prove virtually anything, and results need independent replication.
- Systematic reviews and meta-analyses can reliably synthesise available evidence, but are no better than the studies that they contain.
- Psychiatrists have been over-reliant on the pharmaceutical industry to evaluate new products, and to date have failed to conduct any independent large/mega trials.

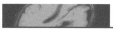 Guidelines

European Union Directive 2001/20/EC on Good Clinical Practice in Clinical Trials (see http://www.mhra.gov.uk for details and current consultation on their implementation)
World Medical Association Declaration of Helsinki. Ethical Principles for Medical Research Involving Human Subjects (Fifth Revision), 2000. http://www.wma.net/e/ policy/b3.htm

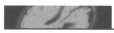 References

Key references

Carpenter WT Jr, Gold JM, Lahti AC et al. Decisional capacity for informed consent in schizophrenia research. Arch Gen Psychiatry 2000; 57:533–8

Chalmers TC, Celano P, Sacks HS, Smith H Jr. Bias in treatment assignment in controlled clinical trials. N Engl J Med 1983; 309:1358–61

Even C, Siobud-Dorocant E, Dardennes RM. Critical approach to antidepressant trials. Blindness protection is necessary, feasible and measurable. Br J Psychiatry 2000; 177:47–51

Moncrieff J, Kirsch I. Efficacy of antidepressants in adults. BMJ 2005; 331:155–7 (response at http:/bonj.brijjournals.com/cgi./eletters/331/7509/155)

Moncrieff J, Wessely S, Hardy R. Meta-analysis of trials comparing antidepressants with active placebos. Br J Psychiatry 1998; 172:227–31; discussion 232–4

Schulz KF, Chalmers I, Hayes RJ, Altman DG. Empirical evidence of bias. Dimensions of methodological quality associated with estimates of treatment effects in controlled trials. JAMA 1995; 273:408–12

Thornley B, Adams C. Content and quality of 2000 controlled trials in schizophrenia over 50 years. BMJ 1998; 317:1181–4

Vastag B. Helsinki discord? A controversial declaration. JAMA 2000; 284:2983–5

Walker AM, Lanza LL, Arellano F, Rothman KJ. Mortality in current and former users of clozapine. Epidemiology 1997; 8:671–7

Zornberg GL, Jick H. Antipsychotic drug use and risk of first-time idiopathic venous thromboembolism: a case-control study. Lancet 2000; 356:1219–23

Further reading

Bedi N, Chilvers C, Churchill R et al. Assessing effectiveness of treatment of depression in primary care. Partially randomised preference trial. Br J Psychiatry 2000; 177:312–18

Edwards IR, Aronson JK. Adverse drug reactions: definitions, diagnosis, and management. Lancet 2000; 356:1255–9

Guyatt G, Sackett D, Taylor DW et al. Determining optimal therapy – randomized trials in individual patients. N Engl J Med 1986; 314:889–92

Hotopf M, Churchill R, Lewis G. Pragmatic randomised controlled trials in psychiatry. Br J Psychiatry 1999; 175:217–23

Kunz R, Oxman AD. The unpredictability paradox: review of empirical comparisons of randomised and non-randomised clinical trials. BMJ 1998; 317:1185–90

Lawrie SM, McIntosh AM, Rao S. Critical Appraisal for Psychiatry. Edinburgh: Churchill Livingstone, 2000

Louis TA, Lavori PW, Bailar JCD, Polansky M. Crossover and self-controlled designs in clinical research. N Engl J Med 1984; 310:24–31

Marshall M, Lockwood A, Bradley C et al. Unpublished rating scales: a major source of bias in randomised controlled trials of treatments for schizophrenia. Br J Psychiatry 2000; 176:249–52

Pocock SJ. Clinical Trials: A Practical Approach. Chichester: John Wiley, 1983

Savulescu J, Chalmers I, Blunt J. Are research ethics committees behaving unethically? Some suggestions for improving performance and accountability. BMJ 1996; 313:1390–3

Index

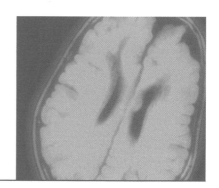

N.B. Page numbers in *italic* denote figures and tables.

aminopyridines *21*
amisulpride 37, *41*
antidepressant 70
  antipsychotic 50
amitriptyline *61, 99*
anandamide 5, 124
Angel Dust *see* phencyclidine (PCP) (Angel Dust)
antagonists 34–5
  effects on agonists *35*
anticholinesterases *see* cholinesterase inhibitors
anticonvulsants 86–93
  antidepressant 92
  antipsychotic 91–2
  anxiolytic 92, 109
  in bipolar disorder 86
  drug interactions *152*
  individual drugs 86–91
  in personality disorders 142
  treatment issues 92
antidepressants 59–72
  α2-adrenoceptor antagonists 69
  in Alzheimer's disease *128*
  anxiolytic 106–7
  in autism 156
  in bipolar disorder 92
  choice of 71
  dementia symptom treatment 136
  dopamine reuptake inhibitors 69
  guidelines 76
  mode of action *57*
  mood stabilisers 69, 92
  noradrenaline reuptake inhibitors (NARIs) 68
  in personality disorders 142
  pharmacology *61*
  phenylpiperazines 67–8
  prophylactic 70
  putative 70
  resistance 71–2
  serotonin hypothesis *57*
  serotonin/noradrenaline reuptake inhibitors (SNRIs) 68, 92
  L-tryptophan *61*, 69
  use of 70–1
  see also selective serotonin reuptake inhibitors (SSRIs); tricyclic antidepressants (TCAs)
antipsychotics 37–55

adverse effects
  akathisia *43*, 44
  cardiac conduction effects 47
  diabetes/metabolic syndrome 46
  dystonia, acute *43*, 43–4
  extrapyramidal side-effects (EPSE) *40, 43*, 43–5, 48, 49
  neuroleptic malignant syndrome (NMS) 45–6
  non-extrapyramidal *47*
  pseudoparkinsonism *43*, 43–4
  reduced in atypicals 48–9
  stroke 47
  tardive syndromes *43*, 44–5
  in Alzheimer's disease *128*
  anticonvulsant 91–2
  anxiolytic 107–8
  atypical 42, 48–54
    atypicality definitions 48
    atypicality mechanisms 48–9
    history 37
    individual drugs 50–4
    mechanisms of action 49
    in schizophrenia 40
  in autism 156–7
  clinical potency *38, 40*
  dementia symptom treatment 136, 137
  dopamine hypothesis of schizophrenia 37–8
  dopamine receptor subtypes *10, 11, 14*
    D2-like receptor occupancy *38, 40*
    drug affinity for *38*
    role of 38–40
  drug interactions *152*
  guidelines 54
  history 37
  indications *41*
  in personality disorders 142
  rapid tranquillisation *146*
  therapeutic actions 40–3
    antipsychotic action 42
    relapse prevention 43
    sedation/tranquillisation 42
  therapeutic range 48
  typical
    chemical classification *41*
    newer type *41*
    older type *41*
anxiety/anxiety disorders
  brain aversion system 96